The Training Courses of Urological Laparoscopy

Ying Hao Sun • Arthur D. Smith
Editors

The Training Courses of Urological Laparoscopy

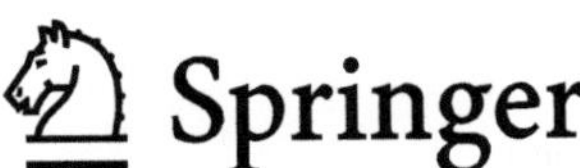

Editors
Ying Hao Sun, M.D.
Department of Urology
Changhai Hospital
Shanghai
China

Associate Editor
Bo Yang, M.D.
Department of Urology
Changhai Hospital
Shanghai
China

Arthur D. Smith, M.D.
Department of Urology
Arthur Smith Institute of Urology
Long Island Jewish Medical Centre
New Hyde Park, NY, USA

ISBN 978-1-4471-2722-2 ISBN 978-1-4471-2723-9 (eBook)
DOI 10.1007/978-1-4471-2723-9
Springer Dordrecht Heidelberg New York London

Library of Congress Control Number: 2012941849

Printed on acid-free paper

Springer is part of Springer Science+Business Media (www.springer.com)

Preface

Since the early 1990s, with the introduction of laparoscopic techniques, laparoscopy has been a rapidly evolving area of urology. Even for more difficult advanced procedure, such as partial nephrectomy and radical prostatectomy, laparoscopy has become an option in hands of skilled surgeons. With the popularity of this technique, residents have been required to develop more skills in less time. However, issues of patient safety, costs, time constraints, and logistics have inevitably limited training opportunities for the novices in the operating room (OR). And most surgical textbooks just provide some standard methods of performing an operation or some surgical tricks and tips. It is more critical to teach residents how to gain enough surgical skills to reduce the complication during the initial stage. And with the increasing use of the laparoendoscopic single-site surgery (LESS) and robotic surgery in the urology, appropriate training programs also need to be established for mastery of these new technologies.

In pursuit of this goal, we sought to provide a special book which is very strong on details of training and will provide a benchmark, a line in the sand. This book takes some experts in laparoscopic urology together from across the world to share their ideas and experience of training, from basic stems in the dry lab through to hints and tricks for problem solving in complex scenarios. Many training models in this book can be referred, which will make the training course easier and more efficient. There is a desire among more and more residents to realize the importance of laparoscopic training and establish the individualized program with the help of this book.

We are grateful that all the contributors completed their assignment in a timely manner to ensure that this book is truly a state-of-the-art reference. I am also grateful for the time, effort, and creativity that each of the contributors put forth on behalf of the book. It has been a pleasure to work with the entire staff of Springer Publishers. Their guidance and expertise were invaluable. I would also like to thank my dear wife for her support related to this project.

Ying Hao Sun, M.D.

Contents

Contributors

Sanket Chauhan, M.D. Department of Urology, Global Robotics Institute, Florida Hospital Celebration Health, Celebration, FL, USA

Rafael F. Coelho, M.D. Departmento do Urologia, Hospital Israelita Albert Einstein, São Paulo, Brazil

Instituto do Câncer do Estado de São Paulo, São Paulo, Brazil

Department of Urology, Global Robotics Institute, Florida Hospital Celebration Health, Celebration, FL, USA

Cardeal Arcoverde, Sao Pãulo, Brazil

Mahesh R. Desai, M.S., FRCS (Edin.), FRCS (England) Department of Urology, Muljibhai Patel Urological Hospital, Nadiad, Gujarat, India

Arvind Prakash Ganpule, M.S. (Gen. Surg.), DNB (Urology) Department of Urology, Muljibhai Patel Urological Hospital, Nadiad, Gujarat, India

Xin Gao, M.D., Ph.D. Department of Urology, The Thirds Affiliated Hospital, Sun Yat-sen University, GhuangDong, GuangZhou, China

Jian Huang, M.D., Ph.D. Department of Urology, Sun Yat-sen Memorial Hospital, Sun Yat-sen University, GuangZhou, GhuangDong, China

Tae Hyo Kim, M.D. Department of Urology, Dong-A University Hospital, Seo-Gu, Busan, Korea

Estevao A.R. Lima, M.D., FEBU, Ph.D. Department of Urology, Hospital of Braga, Life and Health Sciences Research Institute (ICVS), ICVS/3B's - PT Government Associate Laboratory, School of Health Sciences, University of Minho Braga/Guimarães, Portugal

Zeph Okeke, M.D. Department of Urology, Smith Institute for Urology, North Shore – Long Island Jewish Medical Centre, Lake Success, NY, USA

Zhamshid Okhunov, M.D. Department of Urology, Smith Institute for Urology, North Shore – Long Island Jewish Medical Centre, Lake Success, NY, USA

Kenneth J. Palmer, M.D. Department of Urology, Global Robotics Institute, Florida Hospital Celebration Health, Celebration, FL, USA

Vipur R. Patel, M.D. Department of Urology, Global Robotics Institute, Florida Hospital Celebration Health, Celebration, FL, USA

Ananthakrishnan Sivaraman, M.S., MCh, DNB, FRCS (Urol) Department of Urology, Global Robotics Institute, Florida Hospital Celebration Health, Celebration, FL, USA

Arthur D. Smith, M.D. Department of Urology, Arthur Smith Institute of Urology, Long Island Jewish Medical Centre, New Hyde Park, NY, USA

Ying Hao Sun, M.D. Department of Urology, Changhai Hospital, Shanghai, China

Gyung Tak Sung, M.D. Department of Urology, Dong-A University Hospital, Seo-Gu, Busan, Korea

Eugen Yuhui Wang, M.D., Ph.D., FEBU Department of Urology, Clinic for Urology and Andrology, Eskilstuna/Stockholm, Sweden

Centre for Clinical Research Sörmland, Uppsala University, Sweden

Huiqing Wang, M.D. Department of Urology, Changhai Hospital, Shanghai, China

Zhenjie Wu, M.D. Department of Urology, Changhai Hospital, Shanghai, China

Liang Xiao, M.E. Department of Urology, Changhai Hospital, Shanghai, China

Bo Yang, M.D. Department of Urology, Changhai Hospital, Shanghai, China

Chapter 1
The Role of Laparoscopy Training in Urology

Zhamshid Okhunov, Zeph Okeke, and Arthur D. Smith

Abstract The introduction of laparoscopic surgery into urology has led to new training concepts. Reduced depth perception, loss of haptic feedback, restrictive freedom of movement, and requirement of a video-eye-hand coordination are the major concerns of contemporary laparoscopic surgery. Laparoscopic skills and competence are a combination of knowledge, judgment, technical ability, and, particularly important, training. Adequate laparoscopic fellowship training contributes to increased activity in laparoscopic surgery and decreased complication rates. The cost, medicolegal, and ethical issues have made the training in laparoscopic urologic surgery challenging. Surgical simulators (box trainers, VR simulators, animal models, etc.) definitely play an important role not only in learning a procedure but also in maintaining skills and preparing for the management of complications.

Keywords Urology • Laparoscopy • Skill • Training

Z. Okhunov, M.D. • Z. Okeke, M.D.
Department of Urology,
Smith Institute for Urology, North Shore – Long Island Jewish Medical Centre,
450 Lakeville Road, Suite M41, Lake Success, NY 11042, USA

A.D. Smith, M.D. (✉)
Department of Urology, Arthur Smith Institute of Urology, Long Island Jewish Medical Centre,
450 Lakeville Road, New Hyde Park, NY 11040, USA
e-mail: asmith1@lij.edu

Y.H. Sun et al. (eds.), *The Training Courses of Urological Laparoscopy*,
DOI 10.1007/978-1-4471-2723-9_1,

1.1 Introduction

Traditionally, open surgery has been employed in the radical treatment of the genitourinary tract pathology. Currently, patients suffering from urologic malignancies can select from numerous treatment options. The modern urologic surgeon must have a profound knowledge of the disease process and also show a technical proficiency of a variety of surgical procedures, including both open and minimally invasive methods. The introduction of laparoscopic surgery into urology has led to new training concepts. The skill set required to perform laparoscopic surgery is significantly different from one that is required for open surgery. Laparoscopic surgery requires adapting to reduced depth perception, developing a video-eye-hand coordination, and becoming accustomed to utilizing long instruments with diminished tactile feedback. That is why it is not surprising that laparoscopic procedures initially take significantly more time to perform compared to their open surgery counterparts [1–3].

In open surgery, surgeons have direct visual input and are able to utilize various cues such as stereopsis to ascertain depth. In contrast, the flat-screen monitors used in laparoscopic surgery result in a reduction of the depth. It is not entirely eliminated, however, as the monitor still provides some features such as interposition or overlap, lighting, outline, texture, and motion parallax [4]. There have been many investigations performed to evaluate the effect of different viewing conditions, comparing 2D and 3D video systems which restore stereoscopic vision [5–7]. Furthermore, experience and adaptation do not seem to be factors influencing performance with different video systems as researchers cannot demonstrate any superiority of 3D system over 2D system for surgeons who have laparoscopic experience and for those who have none [8]. The experience of the surgeons, tasks performed, and equipments used in these studies were widely varied, and more research is needed to determine the effect of depth perception on surgical performance. In addition to the reduction in depth perception, hand-eye coordination for laparoscopic surgeons is also impaired. Other factors that contribute to poorer hand-eye coordination are location of the monitor, variable amplification, mirrored movement, and misorientation [9, 10]. As such, planar disorientation results in increased navigational difficulties for laparoscopic surgeons which lead to significant decrease in performance [11, 12]. Technical solutions for the compensation of planar disorientation are still in the process of being enhanced and validated.

In laparoscopic surgery, the trocar restricts movement by acting as invariant points. The range of motion is therefore reduced to four degrees of freedom compared to six needed to perform free motion, negatively affecting the surgeon's dexterity [13]. Ergonomic analysis of laparoscopic surgery tasks reveals that there are significant ergonomic problems with the use of laparoscopic instruments, which result in more discomfort for the surgeons. In addition, haptic feedback is reduced in laparoscopic surgery due to the use of long and slender laparoscopic instruments. The role of haptic feedback is of special interest because it is used in important decision-making scenarios such as the discrimination of healthy versus abnormal tissues, identification of organs, and motor control. The investigation of challenges in LS and underlying perceptual factors emphasizes limitations in visual and haptic perceptions as two complex and interconnecting issues involved in LS. Under normal circumstances, the redundancy in the human perceptual modalities enables us to compensate for inadequacies in one modality with cues from other modalities. For instance, the perception of a rough surface may involve visual, auditory, and haptic perceptions, but during laparoscopic surgery, both visual and haptic perceptions are impaired, and there is no auditory perception resulting in a less accurate evaluation.

It is clear from the perceptual limitations and their consequences that laparoscopic surgery requires a different motor and perceptual skill set compared to open surgery and training and significant experience are needed to attain competency. Laparoscopic skills and competence are a combination of knowledge, judgment, technical ability, and, particularly important, training.

The surgical learning curve remains primarily a theoretical concept, and laparoscopic surgery has a steep learning curve associated with a higher complication rate in the beginning of the surgeon's experience. What is the learning curve? The German psychologist Hermann Ebbinghaus first introduced the concept of the learning curve. In his study of memorization, he tested his long-term memory by attempting to memorize a series of nonsense syllables. He realized that the more he repeated the series, the more syllables he could remember, until finally he could recall the whole list. If we want to apply this concept to surgery, we would need to draw a slope, and the definition of the learning curve would be the beginning of the slope. It is still controversial how many procedures are required b y a single surgeon to overcome the technical obstacles and achieve satisfactory performance. The Endourological Society requires at least 40 laparoscopic procedures in one-year period in order for a fellowship to be recognized. But it is problematic to define a certain number of procedures for certification since the number of procedures is relative and depends on various factors and particularly the type of procedure, minor or major. In this regard, a defined number of specific procedures may be more realistic.

1.2 Postgraduate Training

There has been a radical change in urology in the past several years. Minimally invasive surgery has now been accepted as the norm for patient care. This involves a new skill set for those individuals in training and for those who were not trained in their residency. Residency training has been hampered by the reduction of resident work hours, both in Europe and the USA, which has resulted in decreased contact time between patients and residents. The training in the past followed a sequence from observation, assistance, participation under guidance, and finally independence [14]. Technology evolves rapidly, and minimally invasive surgery requires the ability to work with constantly changing equipment, computer, and imaging technology [15, 16]. As a result of this, numerous training courses and workshops have been established to provide basic concepts and even more advanced concepts of laparoscopic surgical skills. The training courses and workshops vary in their specific formats; the vast majority consists of 1 or 2 days of instruction, followed by an in vivo animal-model experience. Alternatively, a longer-term visit from 3 to 6 months at a center with high volume of minimally invasive procedures under the guidance of a mentor certainly provides the best way to acquire the skills of a laparoscopic procedure and to eventually perform the entire procedure in routine practice. Several studies have evaluated the effect of these courses on the surgeon's performance and complication rates. Fisher and colleagues attempted to identify predictors of surgical complication rates in the first 3 and 12 months after a formal course in laparoscopic surgery. They sponsored nine 2-day training seminars in laparoscopic urologic surgery. The course consisted of 8 h of didactic lecture, two live case presentations, 5 h of practicing with laparoscopy simulators, and additional 5 h in a live-animal laboratory [17]. Three months after course completion, participants were mailed a questionnaire. Factors potentially affecting laparoscopic complication rates in the early posttraining period were reevaluated at 12 months to determine their long-term influence. Data from their study confirm both the variability of training requirement for the clinical use of laparoscopy and the impact of no additional training on surgical complication rates. Thirty percent of 3-month respondents stated that following the training course, they performed clinical laparoscopy without additional training. The inverse relationship between laparoscopic complication rates and number of cases performed in both the 3-month and 12-month data is consistent with the differences in rates between additionally trained and non-trained groups. The long-term risk factors for increased laparoscopic complication rates suggest that an association is unclear; it makes intuitive sense that the discourse, feedback, and direction provided by a laparoscopically skilled associate could reduce the primary surgeon's risk for complications. Study suggests that optimal clinical performance of a new skill, as measured by procedural complication rates, cannot be attained during a single postresidency instructional course.

Currently, approximately 10% of graduating chief residents pursue a fellowship, with MIS being one of the most popular. Adequate laparoscopic fellowship training contributes to better outcomes and decreased conversion to open for advanced laparoscopic surgeries. There are currently more than 30 endourology and minimally invasive surgery (MIS) fellowships organized by the Endourological Society and the Society of Urologic Oncology in the United States and internationally. When MIS fellowships were first established, there was no governing body over this postgraduate training experience. The Endourological Society has established criteria to provide accreditation for programs. As the number of fellowship programs seeking certification continues to increase, there is a greater than ever need to define program requirements and to develop a core curriculum that is consistent among approved programs. The movement to establish program requirements and a core curriculum has been prompted by several concerns. First, there is significant variability among programs in the clinical and surgical experience that fellows receive. For example, while some programs through the Society of Urologic Oncology (SUO) concentrate on the management of urological malignancies with mentoring opportunities by leaders in open surgery and provide a good open surgical experience, an adequate minimally invasive surgical experience may be lacking. Conversely, programs through the Endourological Society also concentrate on benign urological disease, and surgical focus is on laparoscopic or robotic surgery while experience with open surgical procedures is limited. In general, as indications for minimally invasive surgery in urologic oncology continue to expand, fellows have benefited from increasing exposure to advanced laparoscopic techniques. Fellows now believe that they will finish training with the laparoscopic skills necessary to treat genitourinary malignancies, and accordingly, they plan to perform more laparoscopic procedures upon completing fellowship training. The surveys of fellowship programs indicate that this impressive increase in fellows' comfort with minimally invasive surgery training is due to a combination of improved competency of the teaching staff as well as a dramatic increase in the number of these procedures performed during the fellowship.

The following question remains: What impact does completion of a minimally invasive surgery fellowship have on fellows' future practice and careers? Several studies sought to determine the former fellows' perception of their fellowship experience and how it affected their current clinical practice. Fellowship-trained, minimally invasive urologists show the best performance statistics with regard to cases performed and complication rates when compared with contemporaries who have undergone alternative training methods. Urologists who were in at least 1-year laparoscopic fellowship training performed on average 25 laparoscopic cases per year [18], compared to only 54% of urologists who participated in short courses who still performed laparoscopic procedures 5 years later. Shay et al. reported that participation in laparoscopic surgery during residency training has been considered a major determining factor in the performance of laparoscopy as a primary surgeon in practice. Similarly, Rane and colleagues reported increased activity in laparoscopic renal surgery in clinical practice following dedicated fellowship training focused on laparoscopic urological surgery.

The role of the mentor is invaluable in creating an effective teaching environment and involves two critical aspects: (a) the surgeon-in-training must participate to acquire part of the skills, landscape, and navigational knowledge necessary for him or her to become a proficient laparoscopic surgeon; (b) also as important, the trainee should play an essential role in the operation he or she assists in, with part of the responsibility in the evolution and outcome of the procedure. These two aspects are related but not at all the same. The first is indeed the role of the trainee with his or her mentor, as the two together form an *apprenticeship*. The second should not be relegated to a master/slave relationship, but rather a *partnership* in which the assistant provides accurate, precise, and adapted vision, anticipating the needs of the operator without leaving the field of attention too quickly or unattended, therefore ensuring the same safety measures as the operating surgeon.

1.2.1 Training Challenges

Widespread acceptance of laparoscopic urology techniques has posed many challenges to training urology residents and allowing postgraduate urologists to acquire difficult new surgical skills. Several factors in surgical training programs are limiting the ability to train residents in the operating room, including limited-hour work weeks, increasing demand for operating room productivity, and general public awareness of medical errors. This has led to the development of a variety of additional tutorials for improving laparoscopic assistant skills including instructional videos, "wet" laboratories, simulators, robotics, pelvic trainers, and peer review or video critiques of task performance. Laboratory or simulator training may also increase familiarity with technique and technology plus operative conduct of actual procedures. Other methods employ using virtual reality to expand the scope of visually realistic multidimensional laparoscopic simulation. Similar multimedia programs enable the assistant/apprentice to view standardized approaches to many procedures. Using these systems, the surgeon can study a variety of techniques to accomplish different laparoscopic objectives. Various types of training tools and simulators have been developed. They are diverse in their platforms and performance assessments.

1.3 Surgical Simulators

1.3.1 Box Trainers

Incorporating training tools into the training paradigm provides the promise of an effective and rapid development of skills. However, these systems range in price from approximately several thousand dollars up to $300,000 per simulator. Thus, it is difficult to promote their widespread use, as they are excessively expensive for common use by urology departments.

Recent efforts to create affordable training boxes resulted in products such as the EZ trainer. Landman and colleagues developed a portable and cost-effective laparoscopic trainer. The advantage of these types of trainers is that they are relatively inexpensive and have a small, compact, and lightweight design to allow storage and portability for home or office. These systems have been developed for widespread use among residents and allow not only an affordable tool for practicing, but the ability to practice at home.

More laptop-based cost-effective systems have been developed for more widespread dissemination. This type of surgical simulator uses real surgical instruments and equipment including video monitors, cameras, and laparoscopes. It is an opaque box that approximates the size of the adult human abdominal cavity. Slits are prefabricated on the anterior surface of the box, through which trocars (access ports) may be placed. An attached flexible arm acts as a camera holder. Laparoscopic instruments are then inserted through the ports and into the box. Various targets are manipulated inside the box, with visual information relayed through a video source and display comparable to that used in most operating theaters. Tactile feedback is limited, as it is in laparoscopic surgery, by the instruments used. The use of real instruments and equipment is clearly the strength of these systems. However, the drills developed lack the face validity offered by other systems; the instruments may be real, but the "tissues" used clearly are not.

Clayman and colleagues developed a new LapED® 4-in-1 silicone model that provides an inexpensive, versatile educational device for learning four reconstructive laparoscopic urologic procedures. This was the first model to address procedure-specific training in four laparoscopic reconstructive urologic procedures. Both content and face validity of this model were evaluated for two of the reconstructive procedures (i.e., pyeloplasty and vesicourethral anastomosis). The estimated cost of a 4-in-1 model is $100 per model. However, by removing the sutures after every exercise, the procedures may be repeated several times on the same model. Based on authors' experience, they were able to use the model for at least 40 vesicourethral anastomoses and pyeloplasties before discarding it for a new one.

1.3.2 Virtual Reality Simulators

Virtual reality (VR) surgical simulators are the latest and most promising innovative development in the area of surgical simulation. Sophisticated computer software has been developed in an attempt to replicate critical skills required for laparoscopic surgery. Many of the VR simulators offer a more believable practice environment than traditional box trainers, hence providing higher face validity. Another advantage of these trainers is that it can be set up to record and save accurate and objective data for individual performance on specific tasks for later assessment. The metrics of most devices can be customized, setting pass/fail criteria. These features present the opportunity for a trainee to practice independently on their own time as part of a structured curriculum.

The performance records make it possible for the educator to evaluate the performance of a laparoscopic task in an easy accessible format, to track the progress of an individual, and to compare a trainee's results to peers and an expert standard. Virtual reality simulators are also available for technically challenging tasks such as laparoscopic radical nephrectomy, transurethral prostatectomy, and cystoscopy. Objective measurements such as the time to complete a task, economy of hand motion, dexterity, and instrument path length can be easily used as assessment tools to document the progress of laparoscopic skills. In an attempt to replicate the biggest advantage of box trainers and make the simulations as real as possible, several VR simulators now offer built-in haptics, or force feedback, as an option on their systems. These systems, while intriguing, have not yet been shown to significantly contribute to training but do significantly contribute to the cost of the devices.

1.3.3 Animal Models

Although box trainers and virtual reality simulators can provide the necessary basic skills training for endoscopic and laparoscopic surgeons, it is necessary to incorporate live-animal or cadaver practice or both to train fully in the complex techniques of laparoscopy and robot-assisted laparoscopy. These simulators involve the use of a live, anesthetized animal. This is the most realistic, nonpatient environment for laparoscopic training. The abdomen in the porcine model is comparable in size to the adult human, with much of the foregut anatomy similar to that of the human. Performing a nephrectomy in this model provides tactile feedback in an environment where technical errors and complications such as bowel perforation or common vascular injury can occur without consequence to a human patient. Likewise, the canine model is frequently used to practice urologic surgery. Animal models also enable trainees to work together as a team on an operation, providing additional insight into setting up an operative case.

As useful as animal labs are, there are many reasons why they are not fully integrated into most surgical curricula. Ethical issues regarding the use of animals for training and studies are not to be discounted, but for most programs, the cost issues are prohibitive. There are substantial costs associated with maintaining specialized facilities and providing appropriate staff. In some institutions, including our own, these facilities have been converted into an inanimate skills training laboratory.

1.4 Conclusion

In conclusion, surgical skill training is undergoing a dramatic transformation. Modern technology and training techniques, combined with external pressures and mandates, are forcing surgeon-educators to rethink previously held principles. Surgical simulators have the potential to be much more than tools for laparoscopy training and evaluation in urology. As the technology constantly develops, the high standards required for appraisal and certification should allow future generations of simulators to also be used for operative planning. An innovative and progressive approach, learning from the experiences in the field of aviation, can provide the foundation for the next century of surgical training. As the technology develops, the way we practice will continue to evolve, to the benefit of physicians and patients. Obviously, it should be recognized that simulators can never replace operating room experience; however, they will undoubtedly help to enhance and complement the current training paradigm in an efficient and objective manner.

While various opportunities exist for training the future urologic oncologist, none have been proven to be ideal. The traditional training pathway including a residency program followed by extensive fellowship training remains invaluable.

References

1. Ganpule AP, Sharma R, Thimmegowda M, et al. Laparoscopic radical nephrectomy versus open radical nephrectomy in T1-T3 renal tumors: an outcome analysis. Indian J Urol. 2008;24:39–43.
2. Lepor H. Open versus laparoscopic radical prostatectomy. Rev Urol. 2005;7:115–27.
3. Porpiglia F, Volpe A, Billia M, et al. Laparoscopic versus open partial nephrectomy: analysis of the current literature. Eur Urol. 2008;53:732–42; discussion 42–3.
4. Shah J, Buckley D, Frisby J, et al. Depth cue reliance in surgeons and medical students. Surg Endosc. 2003;17:1472–4.
5. von Pichler C, Radermacher K, Boeckmann W, et al. Three-dimensional versus two-dimensional video endoscopy. A clinical field study in laparoscopic application. Stud Health Technol Inform. 1996;29:667–74.
6. Hanna GB, Cuschieri A. Influence of two-dimensional and three-dimensional imaging on endoscopic bowel suturing. World J Surg. 2000;24:444–8; discussion 8–9.
7. van Bergen P, Kunert W, Bessell J, et al. Comparative study of two-dimensional and three-dimensional vision systems for minimally invasive surgery. Surg Endosc. 1998;12:948–54.
8. Chan AC, Chung SC, Yim AP, et al. Comparison of two-dimensional vs three-dimensional camera systems in laparoscopic surgery. Surg Endosc. 1997;11:438–40.
9. Breedveld P, Wentink M. Eye-hand coordination in laparoscopy – an overview of experiments and supporting aids. Minim Invasive Ther Allied Technol. 2001;10:155–62.
10. Hanna GB, Shimi SM, Cuschieri A. Task performance in endoscopic surgery is influenced by location of the image display. Ann Surg. 1998;227:481–4.
11. Ellis SR, Menges BM. Localization of virtual objects in the near visual field. Hum Factors. 1998;40:415–31.
12. Guru KA, Kuvshinoff BW, Pavlov-Shapiro S, et al. Impact of robotics and laparoscopy on surgical skills: a comparative study. J Am Coll Surg. 2007;204:96–101.
13. Lenoir C, Steinbrecher H. Ergonomics, surgeon comfort, and theater checklists in pediatric laparoscopy. J Laparoendosc Adv Surg Tech A. 2010;20:281–91.
14. Rosser Jr JC, Murayama M, Gabriel NH. Minimally invasive surgical training solutions for the twenty-first century. Surg Clin North Am. 2000;80:1607–24.
15. Dent TL. Training, credentialling, and granting of clinical privileges for laparoscopic general surgery. Am J Surg. 1991;161:399–403.
16. Society of American Gastrointestinal Endoscopic Surgeons. Guidelines for institutions granting bariatric privileges utilizing laparoscopic techniques. Society of American Gastrointestinal Endoscopic Surgeons (SAGES) and the SAGES Bariatric Task Force. Surg Endosc. 2003;17:2037–40.
17. See WA, Cooper CS, Fisher RJ. Predictors of laparoscopic complications after formal training in laparoscopic surgery. JAMA. 1993;270:2689–92.
18. Cadeddu JA, Wolfe Jr JS, Nakada S, et al. Complications of laparoscopic procedures after concentrated training in urological laparoscopy. J Urol. 2001;166:2109–11.

Chapter 2
How to Improve Your Laparoscopic Skills Quickly

Mahesh R. Desai and Arvind Prakash Ganpule

Abstract An ideal learning curve ascends through laboratory training, attending structured instructional courses, performing surgeries under supervision of a qualified mentor, followed by performance of cases which are properly selected. Various pelvic trainers such as mechanical trainer, hybrid trainer, and virtual reality trainer in the skills laboratory do help the novices to acquire the basic laparoscopic skills and the video eye-hand coordination. Specialized models for individual procedures (urethrovesical anastomosis, donor nephrectomy, pyeloplasty, etc.) can be easily devised, and boost the trainee's confidence and help in troubleshooting just prior to the procedure. Mentoring is a key component of any laparoscopic training program. A trainee can be mentored in ways of instructional courses, videotape, mutual mentoring, supervised clinical training, telesurgical mentoring, and proper case selection; nevertheless, the obstacles with mentoring lie in commitment from both the trainee and the mentoring surgeon.

Keywords Laparoscopy • Learning curve • Mentor • Training

M.R. Desai, M.S., FRCS (Edin.), FRCS (England) (✉)
Department of Urology,
Muljibhai Patel Urological Hospital,
Dr. Virendra Desai Road, Nadiad, Gujarat 387001, India
e-mail: mrdesai@mpuh.org

A.P. Ganpule, M.S. (Gen. Surg.), DNB (Urology)
Department of Urology, Muljibhai Patel Urological Hospital,
Dr. Virendra Desai Road, Nadiad, Gujarat 387001, India

Y.H. Sun et al. (eds.), *The Training Courses of Urological Laparoscopy*,
DOI 10.1007/978-1-4471-2723-9_2, © Springer-Verlag London 2012

2.1 Introduction

The model "see one, do one, and teach one" does not apply to laparoscopy because of the spatial orientation which needs to be developed in a two-dimensional environment and need for dissection with longer instruments. The inherent learning curve that one has to overcome has been quite convincingly noted in a series wherein there was a decrease in the complication rate from 13.3% to 3% after the first 100 cases [1].The need for overcoming this steep learning curve "quickly" warrants a structured mentored approach for training in laparoscopy.

The training in laparoscopy, to blunt the learning curve, typically involves graded learning curve. An ideal learning curve ascends through laboratory training, attending structured instructional courses, performing surgeries under supervision of a qualified mentor, followed by performance of cases which are properly selected.

The key question we will address in this chapter is how an uninitiated "novice" can start doing laparoscopy quickly for urologic indications.

The pillars for proper laparoscopy training are:

(a) Skills laboratory training
  (i) Pelvitrainer or box trainer training
  (ii) Animal model skill acquisition
(b) Mentor supervised clinical training
(c) Case selection in initial cases

2.2 Skills Laboratory Training

Training in skills laboratory is an initial step in training in laparoscopy. The skills laboratory (pelvitrainer and animal models) helps the individual to acquire the necessary hand-eye coordination and adaptation to 3D vision. The various pelvitrainers that are available are [2]:

2.2.1 Mechanical Trainers

On these models the trainees can learn adaptation to restrictive freedom of movement and reduced haptic feedback. They also help in learning the nuances of handling a laparoscope and trocar placement. Basic steps such as dissection, clipping, and cutting can be practiced. These models are comparatively cheap (Fig. 2.1).

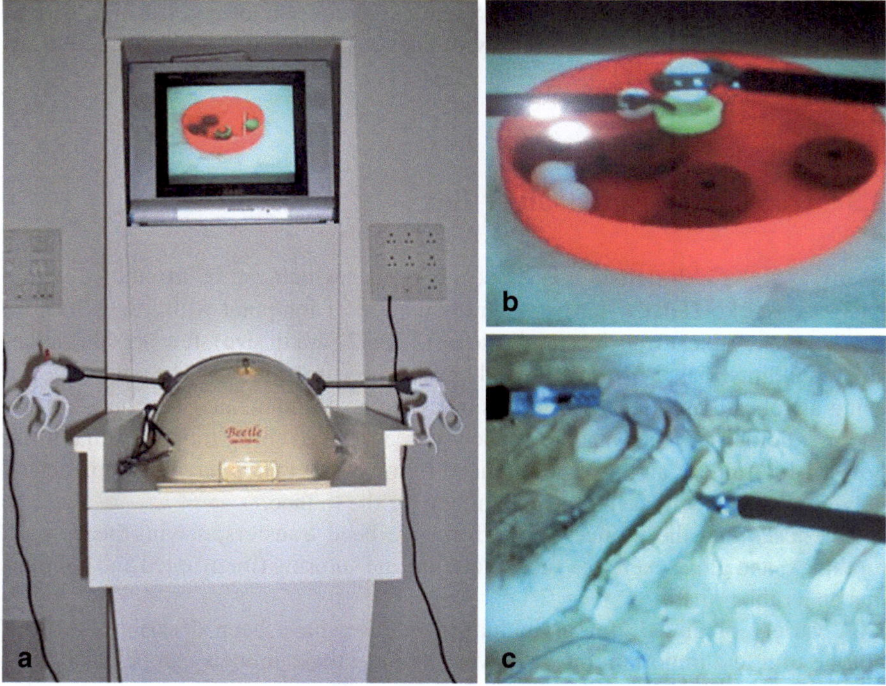

Fig. 2.1 Skills laboratory training on pelvitrainer. (**a**) Simulator for laparoscopy. (**b**) Skills laboratory exercises. (**c**) Knot tying skills on rubber pad

2.2.2 *Hybrid Trainers*

They are similar to mechanical trainers except they receive inputs from a computer. The trainer also gets a tactile feedback.

2.2.3 *Virtual Reality*

These have the capability to manipulate the images and receive a feedback. For beginners the mechanical trainers are the best as they are cheap and can be easily assembled. The trainers can be assembled with the following components, namely, webcam, cardboard box, and desk lamp. The trainee can cut out a task for himself and can score himself on a scorecard.

Standardized programs can be used to assess the baseline laparoscopic skills and track the trainee's progress. The McGill inanimate system for training and evaluation of laparoscopic skills (MISTELS) [3] consists of peg transfer, pattern cutting, ligating loops, and suturing with knots. All these can be performed on an endotrainer box.

2.3 Homemade Endotrainer Box

Beatty et al. have described a laparoscopic trainer which can be assembled with a meager cost of 50 GBP [4]. The assembly requires a computer with free USB port, a webcamera, a clear translucent plastic box (30×20 cm in size), few reusable adhesives, building brick, a 5-mm drill, and laparoscopic instruments. The advantages of using a webcam are that it will act as a "cybercamera man" and has the ability to zoom or defocus. The advantage of such webcam-based cheap trainers is that it can be used by trainees and obviate the need to travel to centers having sophisticated pelvitrainer. This will save time and money for the trainee.

The tasks that the trainee can perform are bead transfers, sewing beads on a toothpick, and glove exercises such as cutting and suturing (interrupted and continuous on a rubber mattress) (Fig. 2.1).

A variety of models for individual procedures have been described. A brief outline of a few important ones is given. Most of these models can be easily prepared and practiced just prior to the procedure. The trainee can practice on this model just prior to the case which will boost his confidence and help in troubleshooting.

2.3.1 Model for Urethrovesical Anastomosis

Two 10-cm segments of pigs' intestine are used to create the model. One segment of the pig's intestine is placed over a syringe and secured to the syringe with 2-0 silk. This represented the bladder portion. The urethral portion is created by placing the other segment of pig intestine over a 15-ml centrifuge tube; this represents the bladder. The whole assembly is kept in a box trainer. Once the anastomosis is completed by the trainee, it can be tested by injecting water with a syringe. A Petri dish below the neoanastomosis quantified the leakage. A study by Boon et al. on this model suggested that test of performance time and postoperative leakage accurately reflected the experience of the surgeon [5]. Similarly, Laguna et al. [6] have shown the construct validity of chicken model in simulation of laparoscopic radical prostatectomy suture. In this study, after partially emptying the abdominal cavity of a cadaveric chicken, the esophagus was intubated with 18 Fr catheter, and the model was placed in a laparoscopic pelvitrainer. The urethrovesical anastomosis can be practiced on this model (Fig. 2.2).

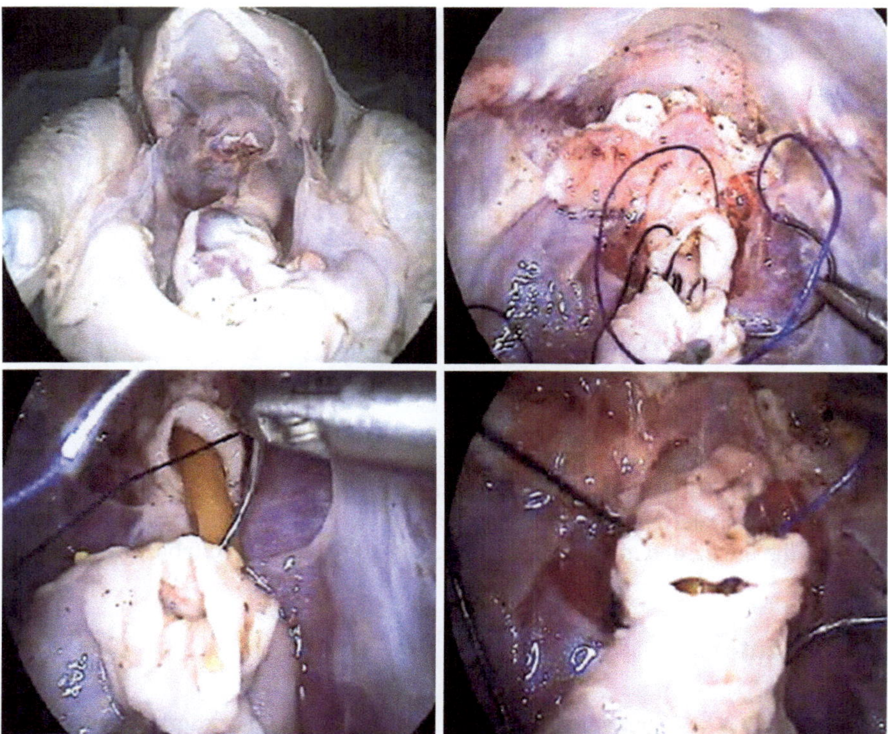

Fig. 2.2 Urethrovesical anastomosis on cadaveric chicken model

2.3.2 Donor Nephrectomy

In a training model by Cavallari et al., the workers performed hand-assisted donor nephrectomy (HALDN) in 10 pigs [7]. They concluded that in vivo training models make it possible to reproduce the positions and operative difficulties encountered in clinical practice. They conclude that this model is a high-fidelity model training procedure that was useful and convenient to achieve skills for HALDN.

2.3.2.1 Laparoscopic Pyeloplasty

Ramchandran and coworkers [8] have devised a model from crop and esophagus of a chicken cadaver (Fig. 2.3). The assembly was placed in a laparoscopic training box. An assessment was done as regards the time required to complete the anastomosis and quality of anastomosis. All the trainees could complete the anastomosis, and there was a significant improvement after the 4th attempt.

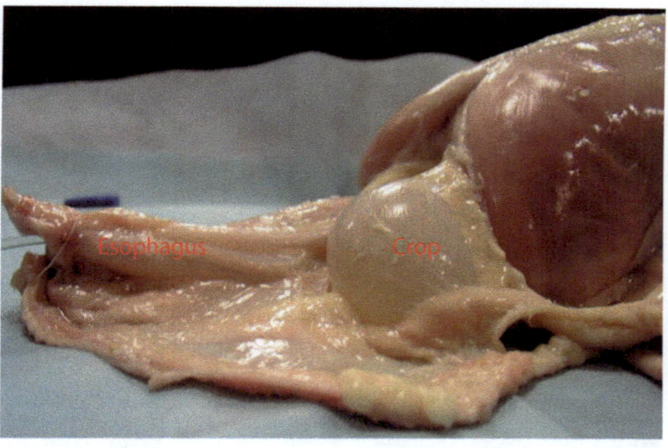

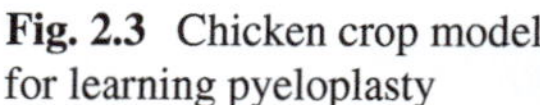
Fig. 2.3 Chicken crop model for learning pyeloplasty

McDougall [9] described a porcine model for training in laparoscopic pyeloplasty. In this model a secondary ureteropelvic junction obstruction was created after ligating the ureter, and after 6 weeks, the enlarged pelvis was suitable for training.

2.4 Mentoring

Mentoring is a key component of any laparoscopic training program. There have been extensive data regarding the usefulness of such training in developing laparoscopic skills. The obstacles with mentoring include commitment from both the trainee and the mentoring surgeon. A trainee can be mentored in the following ways:

2.4.1 Didactic Lectures and Instructional Courses

After attaining basic laparoscopy skills, a brief mentor program simultaneously is advocated to successfully launch the laparoscopic efficiency. There are mini fellowships or a dedicated 2-year endourology or Society of Urologic Oncology fellowship program. The didactic lectures and courses help the trainee to have one-on-one interaction with the trainers and learn the theoretical aspect of the disease and treatment before its application.

2.4.2 Videotape Mentoring

Nakada et al. [10] described the concept of videotape mentoring in teaching advanced laparoscopic techniques. This group of workers demonstrated that videotape critiquing and analysis were beneficial. The uninitiated may benefit by repeatedly viewing the videotapes of operations performed by him or one of his colleagues. A further step in this direction would be reviewing videos of initial cases by the trainee himself. The trainee can identify the pitfalls and the troubleshooting in the cases and improve on them.

2.4.3 Mutual Mentoring

This concept was brought out by Jones and Sullivan [11]. These two authors simultaneously were fellowship trained and performed procedures jointly. The advantage of this procedure as noted by them includes expert camera assistance, a "second opinion" during surgery. This approach benefits two novices at the same time. This approach has the potential to benefit both the parties although it may be geographically restrictive and time-consuming.

2.4.4 Mentored Supervised Clinical Training

This generally is the training in the last stage. The mentored supervised clinical training is also preferably structured. In the initial stage the trainees act as camera driver. This helps in understanding the laparoscopic anatomy and the ergonomics of laparoscopic instrument use. The next step would be performing simple operations such as renal cyst marsupialization, laparoscopic ureterolithotomy, or laparoscopic orchidopexy. All these procedures should be performed under the mentorship of an experienced laparoscopic surgeon.

The mentor should have a keen sense of responsibility and patience for teaching. The mentor gives guidance regarding the anatomic landmarks such as the psoas muscle, aorta and the inferior vena cava, the renal vein, adrenal gland, and the vessels [12, 13]. In pelvic surgeries he also guides regarding the dissection of the space of Retzius.

The mentor can also guide the trainee regarding the tricks of applying a variety of clips and the troubleshooting guidelines in the event of a problem. Such training programs have been developed to develop skills in laparoscopic pyeloplasty and laparoscopic adrenalectomy. The mentored training should be structured for each procedure. The procedure should be divided in steps, and the mentor should take over the case if he feels the case is not progressing or the trainee is not able to handle it. The example of how a procedure for the purpose of mentoring can be divided according to steps is given below:

Laparoscopic Pyeloplasty

1. Trocar placement and dissection of the retroperitoneal space
2. Gerota's fascia incision and mobilization of dilated renal pelvis and upper ureter

3. Trimming of renal pelvis and ureter
4. Corner stitch and excising the stenotic segment with the redundant pelvis
5. Stent insertion and anterior ureteropelvic anastomosis

Laparoscopic Nephrectomy

1. Trocar placement and reflection of the colon
2. Dissection and lifting of the ureterogonadal packet
3. Identification and dissection of the vessels
4. Securing the vessels
5. Dissection of the upper pole
6. Retrieval of the specimen by entrapment in the bag

2.4.5 Telepresence Mentoring

Telesurgical mentoring is an evolving offshoot of telemedicine. This concept involves an experienced surgeon assisting or directing another less experienced surgeon who is operating at a distance [14]. Setup includes real-time transmission of audio and operative images to a central "telesurgical mentor" assisted by 2-way intraoperative interaction. The mentor can guide and teach practicing surgeons new operative techniques utilizing dedicated computer-based image and audio transfer system. This is believed to enhance surgeon's education and decrease the likelihood of complications due to inexperience with new surgical techniques. The goal of this application of telemedicine is to improve surgical education and training for complex laparoscopic urological procedures, with an ultimate aim to improve health-care delivery by widespread availability of urologic surgical expertise. Eventually, surgical telementoring could assist in the provision of surgical training to trainee surgeons with limited experience. It allows novice surgeons with limited formal advanced laparoscopic urologic training to benefit from expert intraoperative advice, simultaneously allaying performance anxiety arising from constant presence of expert surgeon in the vicinity. At the same time, it appears to assist in independent decision making, increasing confidence of operating surgeon, expert help being available as and when needed.

Disadvantages are: requirement of constant involvement of instructor surgeon, and secondly, the telementoring of surgical procedures is currently achieved via a wired infrastructure that usually requires sophisticated videoconference systems along with trained and dedicated IT personnel for troubleshooting and maintenance.

2.4.6 Case Selection

Proper case selection is "key" to success of a laparoscopic surgeon in the initial part of the learning curve (Fig. 2.4). In the initial cases, one should do an axial imaging prior to the procedure; this helps to assess the vascular anatomy as well as helps the

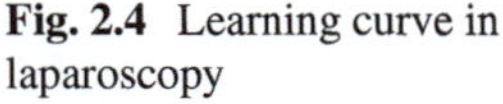

Fig. 2.4 Learning curve in laparoscopy

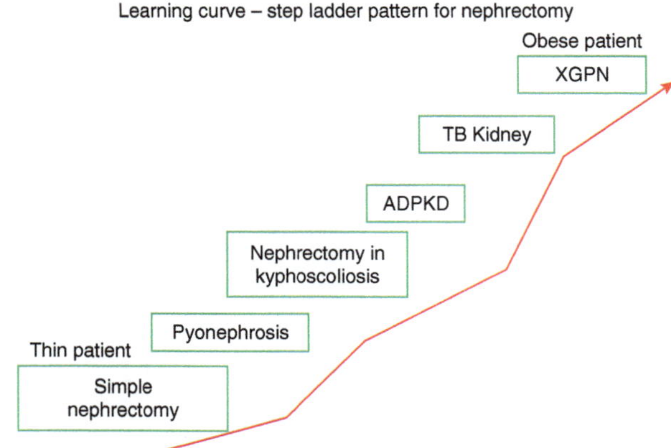

surgeon to predict the possible difficulties he is likely to face during the course of the operation. An improper selection of the case in the initial cases will not only undermine the confidence of the surgeon but will also slow the learning process.

For example, the best case to start with for a nephrectomy would be a thin patient with no adhesions and a single vessel on CT angiography (Fig. 2.5). Although the right side is slightly easier for dissection than the left side, one has to be careful about the vena cava and the short adrenal vein. A thin patient is always desirable than an obese patient from point of view of the morbidity and ease of the procedure. The case selection should be as shown in Figs. 2.4 and 2.6.

2.5 Concluding Remarks

While the Halstedian model of unregulated apprenticeship served trainee surgeon well a century years, the surgical technology of the twenty-first century has increased demands on surgical education. Minimally invasive surgery has radically changed the 3-dimensional visualization and tactile feedback of open surgery. Laparoscopy has further challenged the trainee surgeon by creating a 2-dimensional working environment and reduced tactile sensation.

Being prepared to perform an operation no longer simply means reading the appropriate pages of surgical atlas. Before entering the operating room, the basic skills for minimally invasive procedure such as urological laparoscopy must be developed. This would result in marked improvement of level of care and reduced medicolegal cost. Despite extensive amount of data from the urological literature, the ideal training program in urological laparoscopy remains to be determined objectively. As of today, there is no single-structured and dedicated program for laparoscopic skills training. In view of differing heath-care policies globally, at the moment, the program is fractured. There is a consensus as to what an ideal program should be. It would consist of a combination of inanimate models, animal labs, and clinical exposure under a mentor through fellowship program.

Fig. 2.5 Case selection

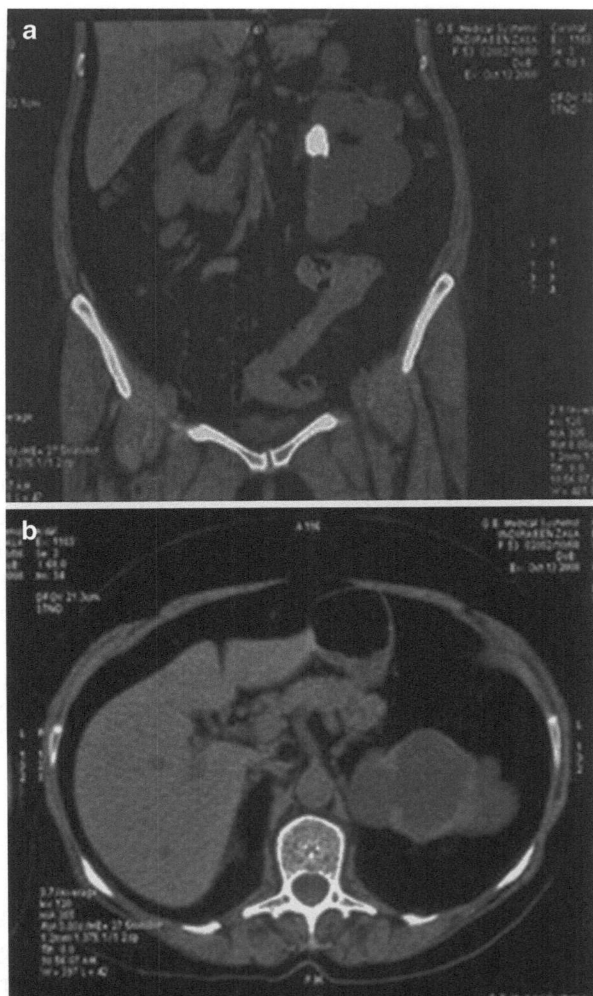

BMI–23 kg/m^2
No perinephric stranding
Single artery and vein
Small non functioning kidney

The ideal training modality requires acquiring basic laparoscopic skills in a dry and wet skills laboratory, simultaneously also acquiring the laparoscopic skills under the guidance of a mentor and then finally doing the procedures independently.

As surgeons, we have a passion for what we do, and we do it to make it the best. To quote Alvin Toffler, "the illiterate of the 21st century will not be those who cannot read and write, but those who cannot learn, unlearn, and relearn." Surgical education requires this same passion and desire for excellence.

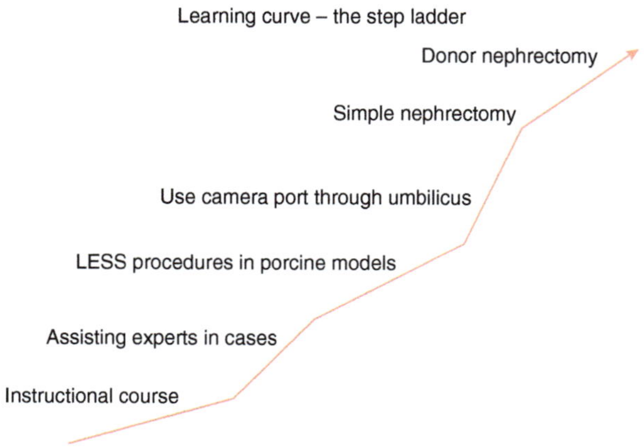

Fig. 2.6 How should one start doing laparoscopy?

References

1. Fahlenkamp D, Rassweiler J, Fornara P, et al. Complications of laparoscopic procedure in urology; experience with 2407 procedures at 4 German centers. J Urol. 1999;162:765–71.
2. Autorino R, Haber GP, Stein RJ, et al. Laparoscopic training in urology critical analysis of current evidence. J Endourol. 2010;24:1377–90.
3. Dausters B, Steinberg AP, Vassiliou M. Validity of the MISTELS simulator for laproscopy training in urology. J Endourol. 2005;19:541–5.
4. Beatty JD. How to build an inexpensive laparoscopic webcam based trainer. BJUI. 2005;96:679–82.
5. Boon JR, Salas N, Avila D. Construct validity of the pig intestine model in the simulation of laparoscopic urerhrovesical anastomosis: tools for objective evaluation. J Endourol. 2008;22:2173–716.
6. Laguna PA, Alacazar AA, Mochtar CA, et al. Construct validity of chicken model in simulation of laparoscopic radical prostatectomy suture. J Endourol. 2006;20:69–71.
7. Cavallari G, Tsivian M, Bertelli R, et al. A new swine training model of hand assisted donor nephrectomy. Transplant Proc. 2008;40:2035–7.
8. Ramachandran A, Kurien A, Patil P, et al. A novel training model for laparoscopic pyeloplasty using chicken crop. J Endourol. 2008;22:725–8.
9. McDougall EM, Elashry OM, Clayman RV. Laproscopic pyeloplasty in the animal mode. JSLS. 1997;1:113–8.
10. Nakada SY, Hedican SP, Bishoff JT, et al. Expert videotape analysis and critiquing benefit laparoscopic skills training of urologists. JSLS. 2004;8:183–6.
11. Jones A, Eden C, Sullivan ME. Mutual mentoring in laparoscopic urology-a natural progression from laparoscopic fellowship. Ann R Coll Surg Engl. 2007;89:422–5.
12. Zhang Xu, Zhang GX, Wang B-J, et al. A multimodality training program for laparoscopic pyeloplasty. J Endourol. 2009;23:307–11.
13. Zhang Xu, Wang B-J, Ma X, et al. Laparoscopic adrenalectomy for beginners without open counterpart experience, initial results under staged training. Urology. 2009;73:1061–5.
14. Lee BR, Bishoff JT, Janetschek G, et al. A novel method of surgical instruction: international telementoring. World J Urol. 1998;16:367–70.

Chapter 3
The Basic Laparoscopic Skills Training Module

Ying Hao Sun, Huiqing Wang, and Bo Yang

Abstract Technical skill is one of the essential competencies of a surgeon, which was developed in clinical work according to traditional surgical training systems. While considering the patient safety, costs, time constraints and logistics, and the characteristic of laparoscopic surgery, training programs outside the operating room have been introduced and developed within the modern surgical educational systems. The basic skills should be mastered in laparoscopic surgery including depth perception, bimanual dexterity, and moving efficiency. In this chapter, we emphasize on detailing the training models and procedures designed to develop the above skills.

Keywords Dry lab • Laparoscopy • Basic skill • Training • Model

3.1 Introduction

Surgeon competency traditionally includes specific knowledge, surgical judgment, and technical skills. Gaining a sound judgment represents the most difficult component among others, implying the need of a long-term training under the guidance of a dedicated mentor. Adequate surgical knowledge can be currently gained by using different educational tools, such as textbooks, multimedia materials, and also internet-based resources. As for technical skills, according to traditional surgical training systems, the trainee is expected to be involved in a supervised clinical setting in order to naturally develop them.

However, issues to patient safety, costs, time constraints, and logistics have inevitably limited training opportunities for the novices in the operating room (OR).

Y.H. Sun, M.D. (✉) • H. Wang, M.D. • B. Yang, M.D.
Department of Urology, Changhai Hospital,
168 Changhai Road, Shanghai 200433, China
e-mail: sunyh@medmail.com.cn

Y.H. Sun et al. (eds.), *The Training Courses of Urological Laparoscopy*,
DOI 10.1007/978-1-4471-2723-9_3,

Thus, training programs outside the OR have been introduced and developed within the modern surgical educational systems.

Compared with open surgery, laparoscopic surgery carries some significant challenges as related to use of elongated instruments (and "fulcrum effect"), decreased tactile feedback, and 2-dimensional visualization [1–4].

Therefore, the need of developing the requisite skills becomes even more critical before landing to the OR for human applications in order to minimize the likelihood of complication [2, 5, 6].

These skills should include depth perception, bimanual dexterity, and moving efficiency, according to the Global Assessment of Laparoscopic Skills system developed by the McGill University. In a controlled laboratory environment, the novice surgeon can gain these pivotal skills by reasonable training courses and specialized training tools [7–11].

Herein, we describe a training module specifically designed for acquisition of basic laparoscopic skills, including camera navigation, eye-hand coordination, and suturing competence.

3.2 Laparoscopic Camera Navigation Skills

3.2.1 Learning Objectives

- To understand the difference between the 0 and 30 degree laparoscope in terms of operative field visualization
- To gain ability in adjusting the focus and in obtaining white balance of the camera
- To understand how to get steady images in different orientations when using a 30 degree laparoscope

3.2.2 Station Setup

- Semicircular-shaped simulator (Fig. 3.1)
- Laparoscopic camera system (Storz)
- 0 and 30 degree scopes
- Two dice (Fig. 3.2)

3.2.3 Description of the Training Procedure

The navigation task is performed according to the following standard operative steps:

- Step 1: Throw two dice into the box trainer.
- Step 2: Adjust the focus and the white balance of 0 degree scope.

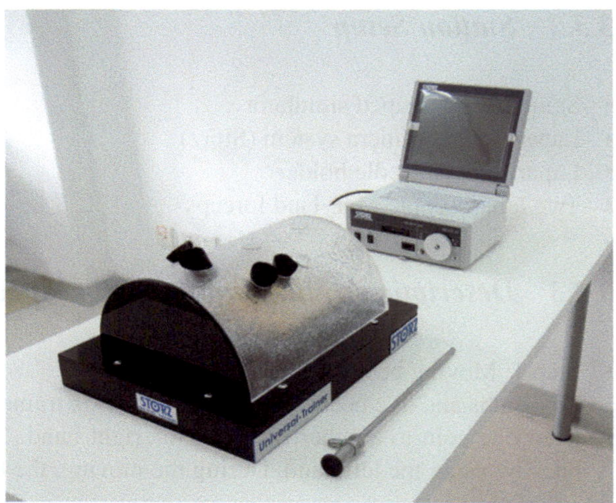

Fig. 3.1 Semicircular-shaped simulator

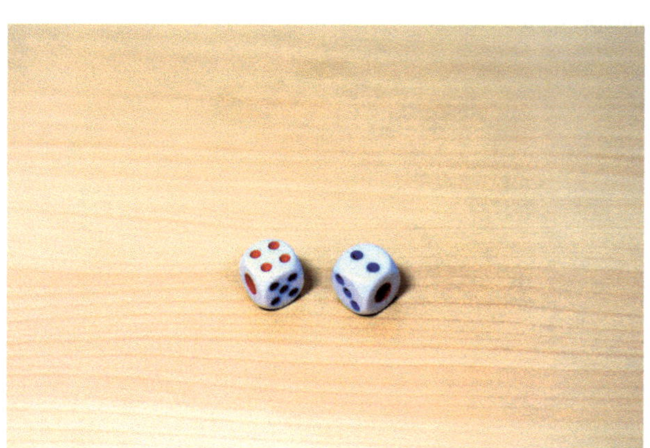

Fig. 3.2 The dice for training

- Step 3: See and record the number of the surface of two dice (Fig. 3.3).
- Step 4: Switch to 30 degree scope, to adjust the focus and to white balance.
- Step 5: See and record the number of two dice.

3.3 Basic Laparoscopic Eye-Hand Coordination Skills

3.3.1 Learning Objectives

- To adapt to elongated laparoscopic instruments
- To develop depth perception during 2-dimensional visualization
- To acquire bimanual dexterity

3.3.2 Station Setup

- Semicircular-shaped simulator
- Laparoscopic camera system (Storz)
- Laparoscopic needle holder
- Two laparoscopic Maryland forceps

3.3.3 Description of the Training Procedure

- Step 1: Moving beans (Fig. 3.4)
  Two coins and five beans are placed in the box trainer. The beans are transferred from one coin to another by using the right hand. Hence, each bean is moved back by using the left hand. During the moving, the beans cannot be dropped.

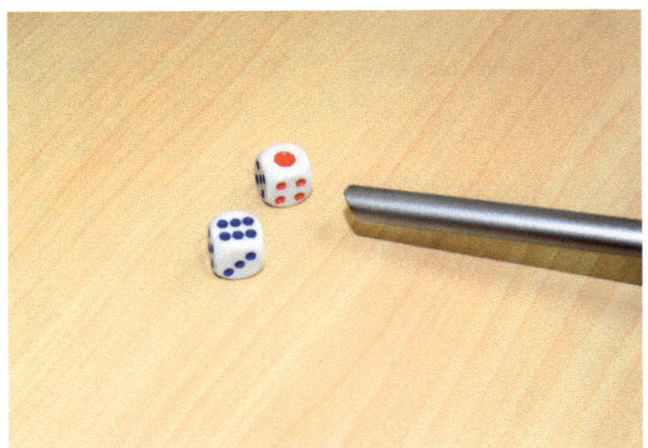

Fig. 3.3 Recording the number on the dice

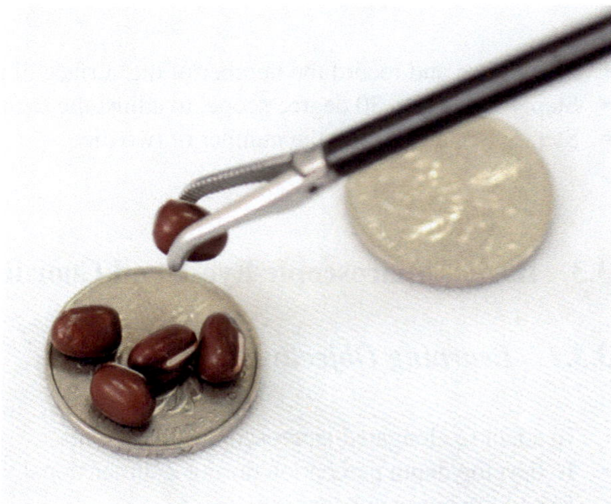

Fig. 3.4 Moving beans

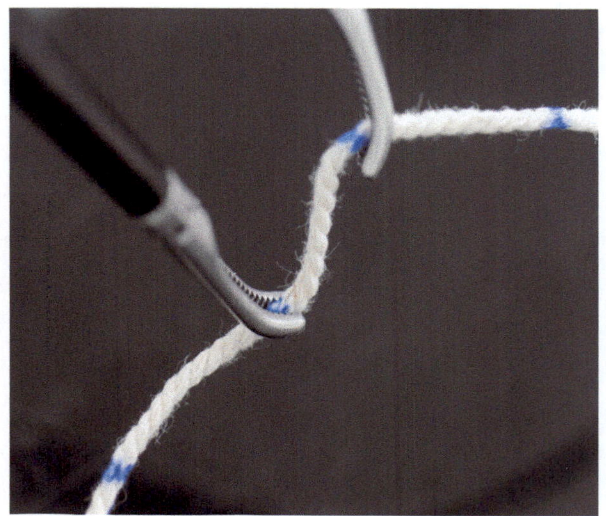
Fig. 3.5 Moving ropes

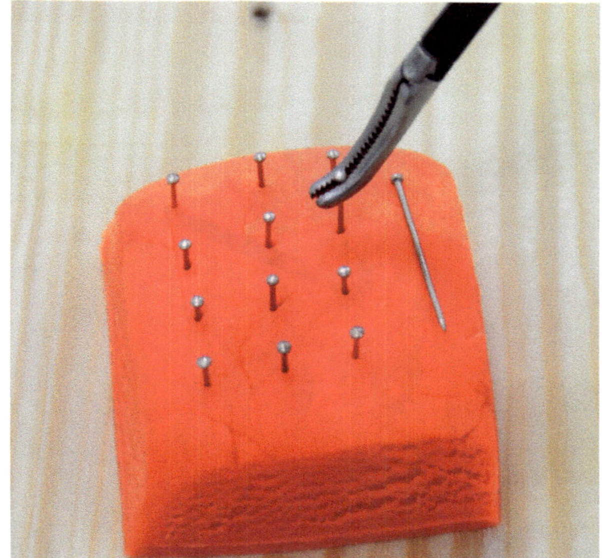
Fig. 3.6 Removing needles

- Step 2: Moving ropes (Fig. 3.5)
  A 20 cm rope is marked every 1 cm. The Maryland forceps is used to move the rope one mark by one mark from one end to the other end, then back in the opposite direction.
- Step 3: Removing needles (Fig. 3.6)
  Twelve needles are pulled out from the plasticine one by one.

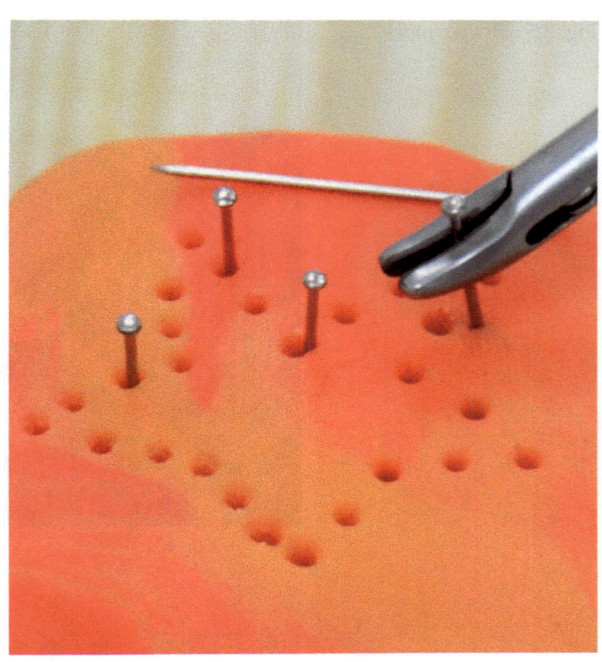

Fig. 3.7 Inserting needles

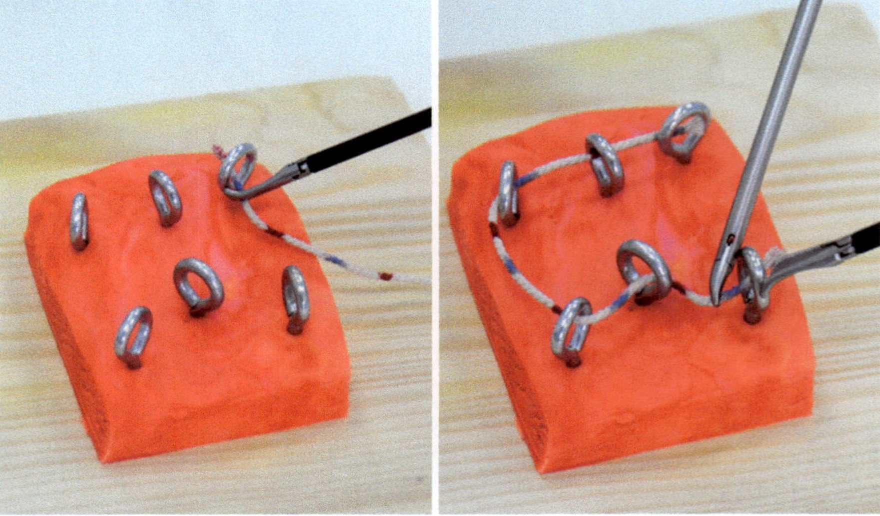

Fig. 3.8 Passing rings

- Step 4: Inserting needles (Fig. 3.7)
  After drawing a star shape on the plasticine with a toothpick, insert the needles into these holes ($n = 26$) by using the needle drive.

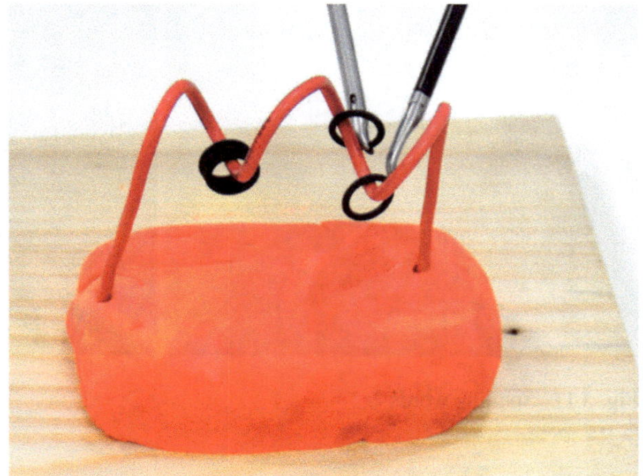

Fig. 3.9 Moving rings

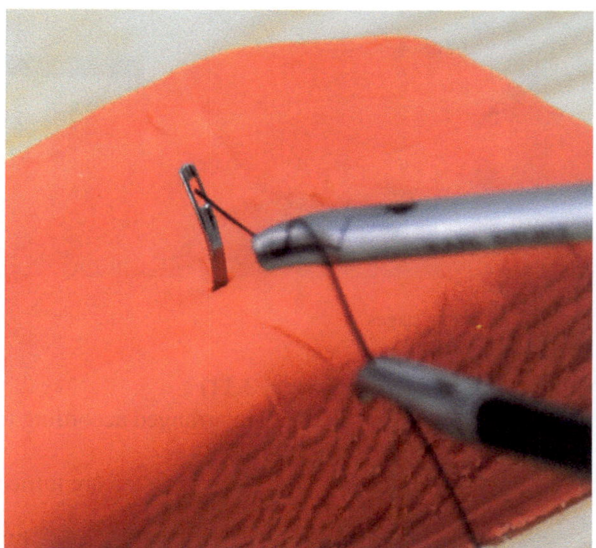

Fig. 3.10 Wearing the eye of needle

- Step 5: Passing rings (Fig. 3.8)
  Six metal ring screws are placed into the plasticine with different heights and directions. Then, a rope is passed through every ring by using two laparoscopic instruments.
- Step 6: Moving rings (Fig. 3.9)
  Six rubber rings are moved through the spiral metal pole from one end to another end.
- Step 7: Wearing the eye of needle (Fig. 3.10)
  Fix the needle in the plasticine, then pass the thread through the eye of the needle ten times.

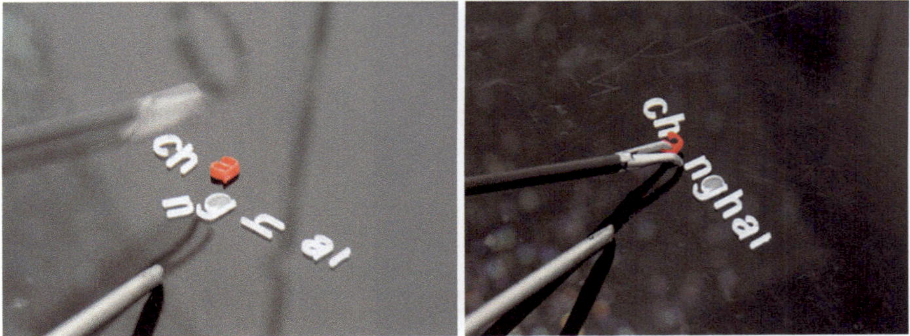

Fig. 3.11 Spelling words

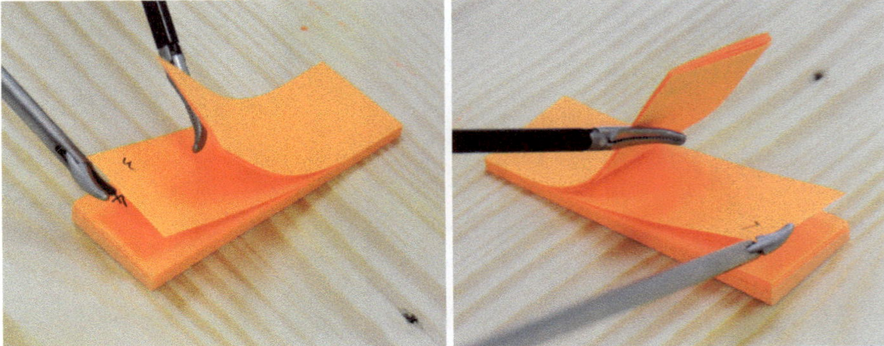

Fig. 3.12 Turning pages

- Step 8: Spelling words (Fig. 3.11)
  The scrambled eight letters are arranged according to the "changhai" sequence.
- Step 9: Turning page (Fig. 3.12)
  Pages of the notes from number one to ten are turned by using two laparoscopic instruments.

3.4 Laparoscopic Suturing Skills

3.4.1 Learning Objectives

- To choose different methods of holding the needle
- To adequately direct the needle
- To tie different knots using laparoscopic instruments

3.4.2 *Station Setup*

- Semicircular-shaped simulator
- Laparoscopic camera system (Storz)
- Two laparoscopic needle drive
- Laparoscopic scissors
- Laparoscopic Maryland forceps
- 2-0 Vicryl suture (7-cm length)

3.4.3 *Description of the Training Procedure*

- Step 1: Changing the direction of the needle point (Fig. 3.13)
  A suture is placed into the box trainer. Then, the suture is grasped at 1 cm away from the needle end with the right hand. Holding the needle point with the left hand, retract the suture with the right hand to adjust the needle point in the 3, 6, and 9 o'clock directions. After putting the needle on the floor, the exercise is repeated three times.
- Step 2: Interrupted suture in different directions (Fig. 3.14)
  A foam is fixed on the floor of the box trainer, and anticipated points for the suture are marked. Then, the 2-0 Vicryl is used to place interrupted sutures in 3, 6, and 9 o'clock positions. One surgical knot and one square knot are tied.
- Step 3: The "U-shape" continuous suture (Fig. 3.15)
  A "U-shape" continuous suture is completed by passing through ten marks on the foam.

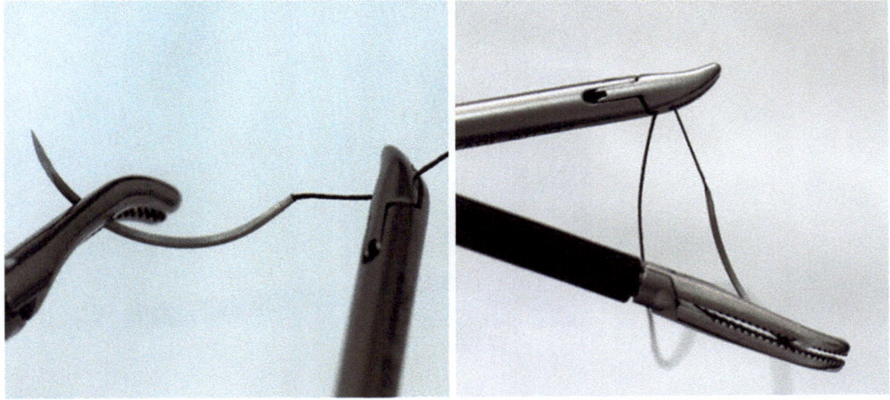

Fig. 3.13 Changing the direction of the needle point

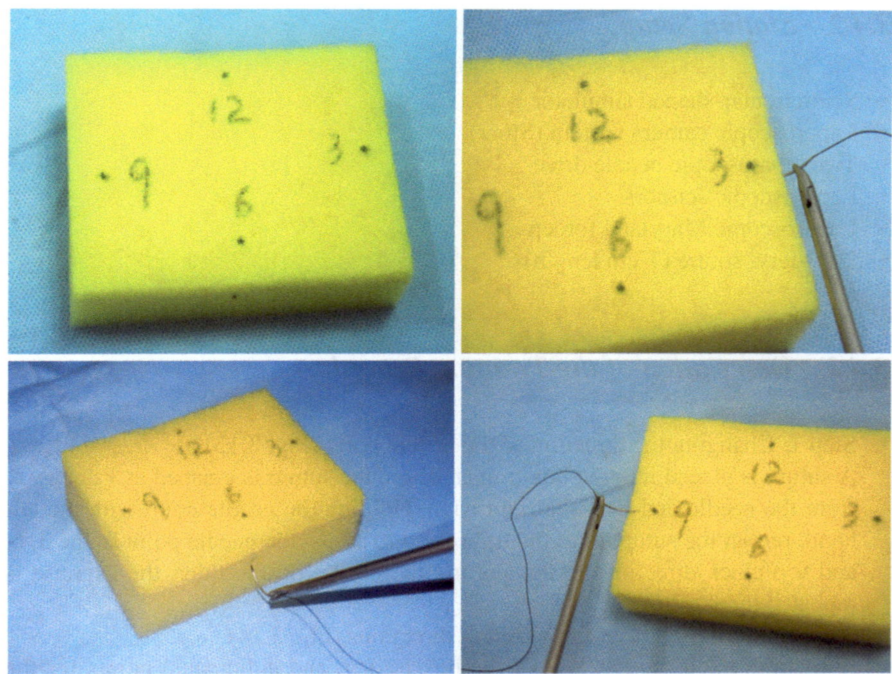

Fig. 3.14 Interrupted suture in different directions

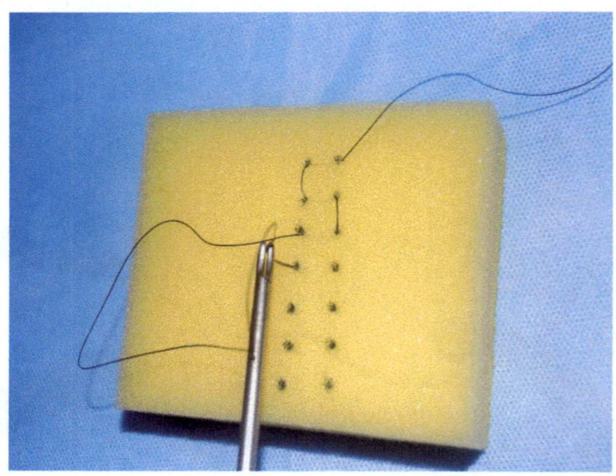

Fig. 3.15 The "U-shape" continuous suture

- Step 4: The ligation of the "Santorini plexus" (Fig. 3.16)
  A roll foam is put on the floor of the box trainer and held with the right hand. The needle is passed through the marks of the roll foam from right to left side, and one surgical and two square knots are tied.

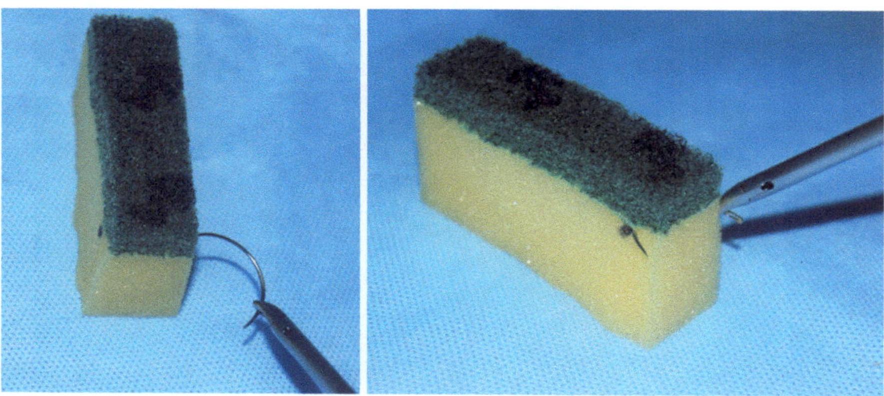

Fig. 3.16 The ligation of the "Santorini plexus"

References

1. Kobayashi SA, Jamshidi R, O'Sullivan P, et al. Bringing the skills laboratory home: an affordable webcam-based personal trainer for developing laparoscopic skills. J Surg Educ. 2011;68:105–9.
2. Jayaraman S, Trejos AL, Naish MD, et al. Toward construct validity for a novel sensorized instrument-based minimally invasive surgery simulation system. Surg Endosc. 2011;25:1439–45.
3. Awtrey CS, Fobert DV, Jones DB. The Simulation and Skills Center at Beth Israel deaconess medical center. J Surg Educ. 2010;67:255–7.
4. Hull L, Kassab E, Arora S, et al. Increasing the realism of a laparoscopic box trainer: a simple, inexpensive method. J Laparoendosc Adv Surg Tech A. 2010;20:559–62.
5. Stefanidis D, Acker CE, Greene FL, et al. Performance goals on simulators boost resident motivation and skills laboratory attendance. J Surg Educ. 2010;67:66–70.
6. Reiley CE, Lin HC, Yuh DD, et al. Review of methods for objective surgical skill evaluation. Surg Endosc. 2010;25:356–66.
7. Edelman DA, Mattos MA, Bouwman DL. FLS skill retention (learning) in first year surgery residents. J Surg Res. 2010;163:24–8.
8. Bokhari R, Bollman-McGregor J, Kahoi K, et al. Design, development, and validation of a take-home simulator for fundamental laparoscopic skills: using Nintendo Wii for surgical training. Am Surg. 2010;76:583–6.
9. Vassiliou MC, Dunkin BJ, Marks JM, et al. FLS and FES: comprehensive models of training and assessment. Surg Clin North Am. 2010;90:535–58.
10. Ali MR, Mowery Y, Kaplan B, et al. Training the novice in laparoscopy. More challenge is better. Surg Endosc. 2002;16:1732–6.
11. Aggarwal R, Moorthy K, Darzi A. Laparoscopic skills training and assessment. Br J Surg. 2004;91:1549–58.

Chapter 4
The Advanced Laparoscopic Skills Training Module

Ying Hao Sun, Liang Xiao, and Bo Yang

Abstract Key steps of laparoscopic reconstruction procedures are based on effective anastomotic or reconstructive techniques, which include radical prostatectomy, pyeloplasty, ureteral reimplantation, and partial nephrectomy. Meticulous suturing skills, adequate exposure of the operative field, and accurate camera navigation which are essential to the success of the above three procedures can be developed by undergoing an intensive advanced training. In this chapter, details of the making of the training models and training procedures designed for the above three procedures are well described. Besides, the "anatomizing the orange" model is also described.

Keywords Dry lab • Urology • Laparoscopy • Advanced skill • Training • Reconstructive model

4.1 Introduction

Undoubtedly, laparoscopic reconstructive procedures are the advanced urological surgeries with a steep learning curve and relative high complication, mainly including radical prostatectomy, pyeloplasty, ureteral reimplantation, and partial nephrectomy. Good anastomosis or reconstruction is the key point of the surgery, which needs more meticulous suturing skill, more reasonable exposure, and more accurate camera navigation [1, 2]. The trainee should progress to the new level by intensive training on these key steps [3–5]. So, we designed three kinds of the targeted reconstructive training model for this "dry lab" module [6, 7]. Meanwhile, the

Y.H. Sun, M.D. (✉) • L. Xiao, M.E. • B. Yang, M.D.
Department of Urology, Changhai Hospital,
168 Changhai Road, Shanghai 200433, China
e-mail: sunyh@medmail.com.cn

Y.H. Sun et al. (eds.), *The Training Courses of Urological Laparoscopy*,
DOI 10.1007/978-1-4471-2723-9_4, © Springer-Verlag London 2012

anatomizing the orange model has proven its value, which can enrich the training program and provide more training of two-handed maneuvers and precise handling skills [8]. In this module, we will describe in detail how to obtain the advanced laparoscopic skills and close to the live animal lab.

4.2 The Training Model of Dismembered Pyeloplasty

4.2.1 Objectives

To understand the basic steps of the retroperitoneum dismembered pyeloplasty and practice the meticulous suturing skills

4.2.2 Station Setup

Semicircular-shaped simulator (Fig. 4.1)
Laparoscopic camera system (Storz)
One laparoscopic needle holder
One pair of laparoscopic scissors
One pair of laparoscopic Maryland forceps

4.2.3 How to Make the Training Model

The maneuvering space in the retroperitoneum was simulated by five boards. Two laterally placed movable boards were fixed by detachable hinges to the base frame. The fixation rod was placed in the lateralmost keyhole.

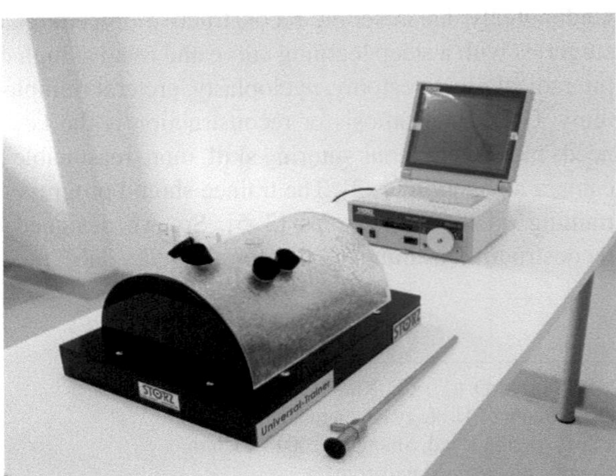

Fig. 4.1 Semicircular-shaped simulator

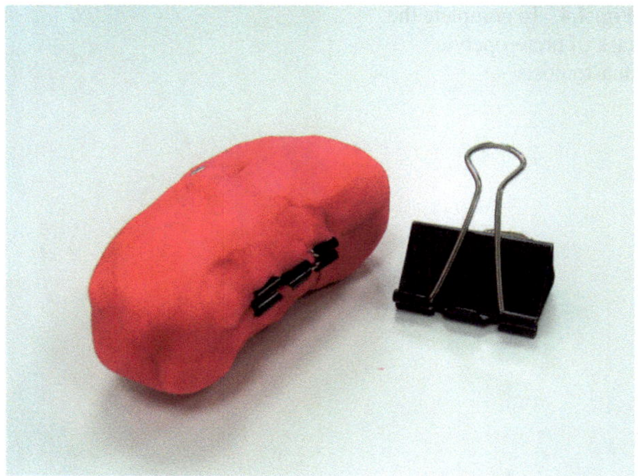

Fig. 4.2 Model of the "kidney"

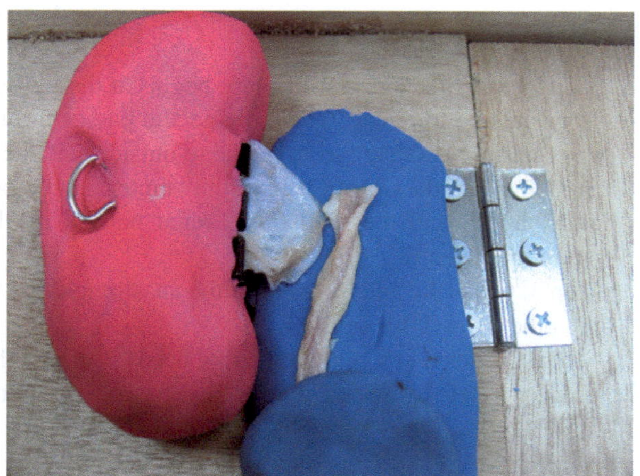

Fig. 4.3 Model of the "renal pelvic" and the "ureter"

The kidney model was made of plastic clay (length-width-height: 10-6-6 cm separately), and a metal clip was imbedded into the middle part (Fig. 4.2). Then a carp swim bladder was fitted to the kidney by the clip to simulate the dilated pelvis. The model ureter was composed of a 10-cm-long porcine ureter (Fig. 4.3).

4.2.4 Description of the Training Procedure

The "ureteropelvic" anastomosis was performed according to the standard operation steps.

Step 1: The "renal pelvis" is excised from its lateral side, and the "ureter" is spatulated longitudinally for 1 cm (Fig. 4.4).

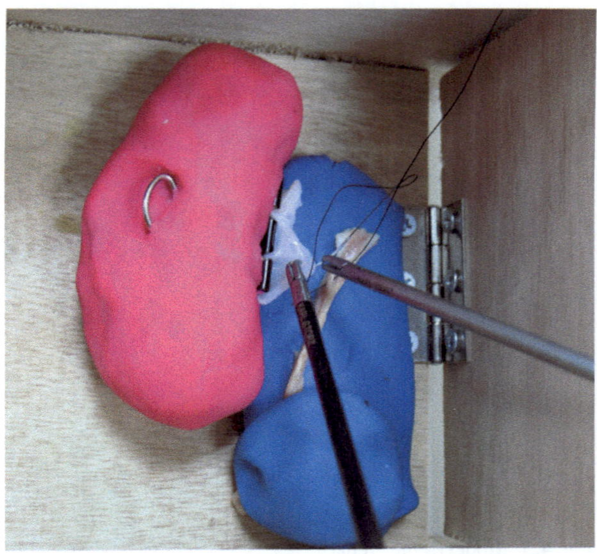

Fig. 4.4 To complete the task of ureteropelvic anastomosis

Step 2: The first Vicryl 4-0 suture begins at the lowest position of "renal pelvis" from outside to inside. Then, the needle passes through the "ureter" wall at the apex of the "V" shape from inside to outside. Tie the first suture.
Step 3: Place the needle behind the "ureter" and close the posterior wall of the anastomosis and the redundant "renal pelvis" by the running suture. Tie the suture at the end.
Step 4: Close the anterior wall of the anastomosis by the interrupted suture using the other Vicryl 4-0 suture.
Step 5: Water is injected with a fine needle through the wall of the sutured swim bladder to test for watertightness and for patency of the anastomosis.

4.3 The Training Model of the Vesicourethral Anastomosis

4.3.1 Objectives

To understand the sequence of the vesicourethral anastomosis and practice meticulous suturing skills

4.3.2 Station Setup

Semicircular-shaped simulator
Laparoscopic camera system (Storz)
Two laparoscopic needle holders
One pair of laparoscopic scissors
One pair of laparoscopic Maryland forceps

4.3.3 *How to Make the Training Model*

Three wooden bars were conjunct together by hinges to simulate the pelvic cavity. Two of them sized 15×5×3 cm while the one in the middle sized 8×5×3 cm with a 10-mm orifice to pass through a simulating urethra. The angles of these bars could be adjusted to simulate various structures of the pelvic cavity as required.

The urethra was simulated with chicken intestines, where an F18 catheter could be inserted to act as sound. And the bladder was simulated with pig intestines which were fixed on the back with pins. An orifice (1 cm in diameter) was created on the opposite side of mesentery to form bladder neck (Fig. 4.5).

4.3.4 *Description of the Training Procedure*

Step 1: Two 3-0 poliglecaprone 25 sutures on RB-1 or SH needles are used for the anastomosis. Each suture is cut to 7 in. in length, and their ends tied together to create a double-armed suture with a total length of 12 in. One sutures by taking a bite outside-in on the bladder at the 7 o'clock position, followed by an inside-out throw at the corresponding position on the urethral stump.

Step 2: After two or three throws have been completed with the first suture, two throws through the bladder and urethra are performed using the other suture, starting at 5 o'clock and progressing slightly counterclockwise.

Step 3: Suturing resumes with the first suture arm, progressing clockwise to approximately the 12 o'clock position. The other suture then completes the anastomosis, proceeding counterclockwise until the two arms of the suture are juxtaposed on the urethral side and a knot is tied (Fig. 4.6).

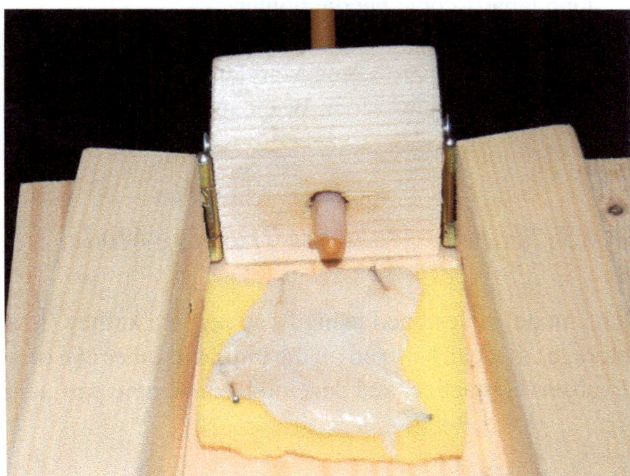

Fig. 4.5 Model of the "urethra" and "bladder"

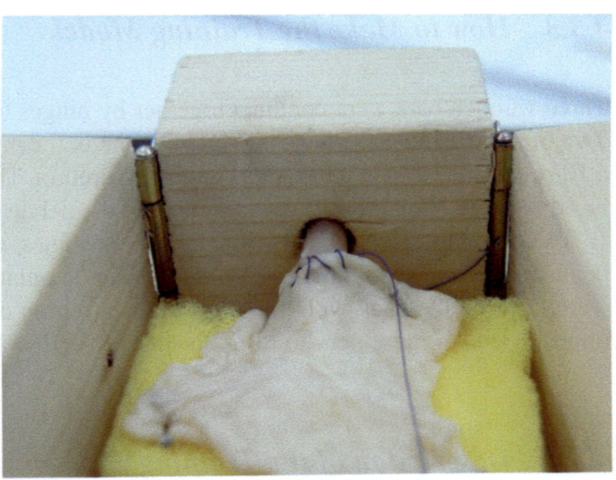

Fig. 4.6 To complete the task of vesicourethral anastomosis

4.4 The Training Model of Partial Nephrectomy

4.4.1 Objectives

To understand the basic reconstructive steps of the partial nephrectomy and practice how to close the renal defect

4.4.2 Station Setup

Semicircular-shaped simulator
Laparoscopic camera system (Storz)
One laparoscopic needle holder
One pair of laparoscopic scissors
One pair of laparoscopic Maryland forceps
One 10-mm hem-o-lock Weck applier

4.4.3 How to Make the Training Model

The model is designed using fresh porcine kidney (less toughness after long frozen storage) that can be fixed on the unfolded inner cap of a metallic box to help trainees to observe, practice, and develop laparoscopic partial nephrectomy skills. The inner

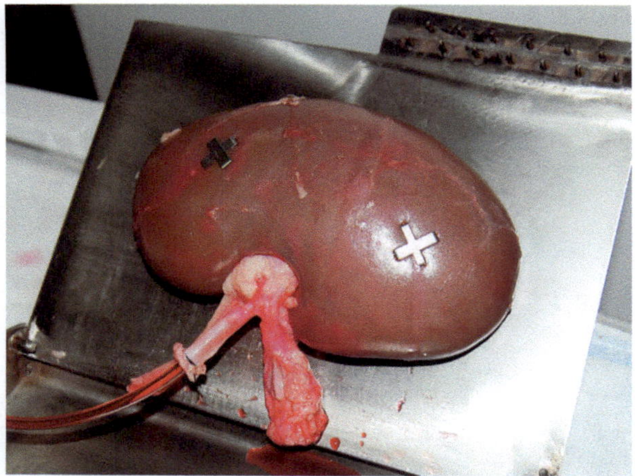

Fig. 4.7 The model of partial nephrectomy

cap of the box, which has been specially designed, had several pins on the flange of one side and small holes in the middle of the cover plate, which is designed for fixing and positioning the porcine kidney. The main body of the box is used as a water trough.

The porcine kidney is procured from a butcher; a section of blood vessels and ureter from the renal hilum has been previously requested to be reserved. Staples can be inserted into the renal parenchyma as a sign of tumor locations. Typically, when the renal artery is infused with red-dyed water stored above in a 3-L bag, the outflow from the renal vein can be seen after some seconds (Fig. 4.7).

4.4.4 Description of the Training Procedure

Partial nephrectomy is performed according to the standard operation steps.

Step 1: The marked "renal tumor" is excised following standard oncological principles (1 cm margin), with the scissors in the right hand and the aid of the forceps in the left hand for providing countertraction. The depth of the renal defect is about 1.5 cm to expose the collecting system. The renal artery needs an unremitting infusion during the procedure (Fig. 4.8).

Step 2A: For the traditional closure method, the collecting system is closed by the Vicryl 3-0 suture in the running method. Then, the renal parenchyma is closed by the Vicryl 1-0 suture in the "8" shape method (Fig. 4.9).

Step 2B: For the knotless closure method, the needle with Vicryl 3-0 suture, tying the Weck clip at the end, passes the renal parenchyma from outside to

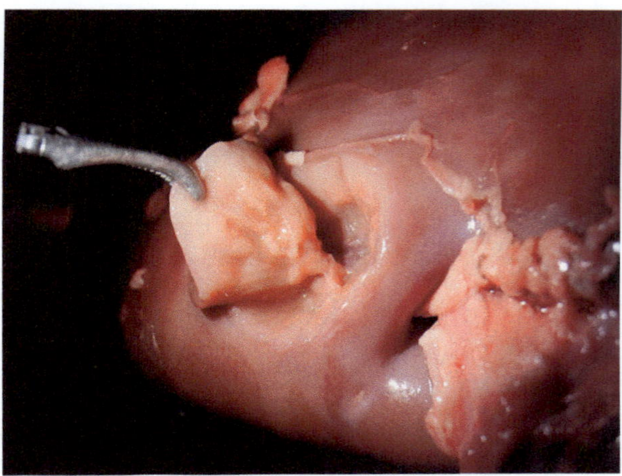

Fig. 4.8 Spherical renal parenchyma excision

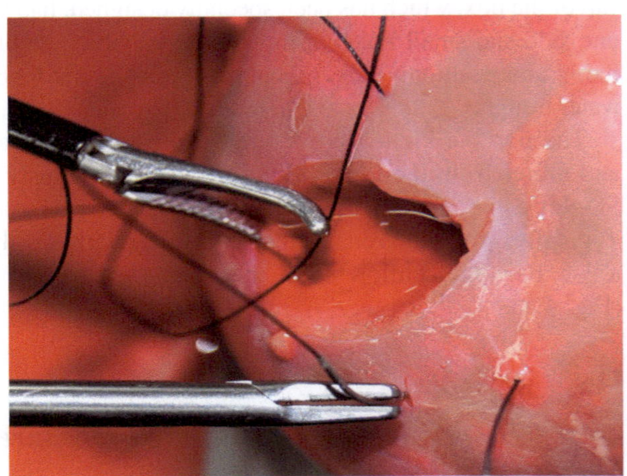

Fig. 4.9 Suturing the bed of resection

inside and closes the collecting system in the running method. Then the needle is pushed out of the renal parenchyma from the other side. The Weck clip is slided to secure the suture. At last, the Vicryl 1-0 suture with the Weck clip at the end is used to close the renal parenchyma in the running method. After every stitch, the Weck clip is used to secure the suture.

Step 3: At the end of the closure, open the renal artery and test the water tightness (Fig. 4.10).

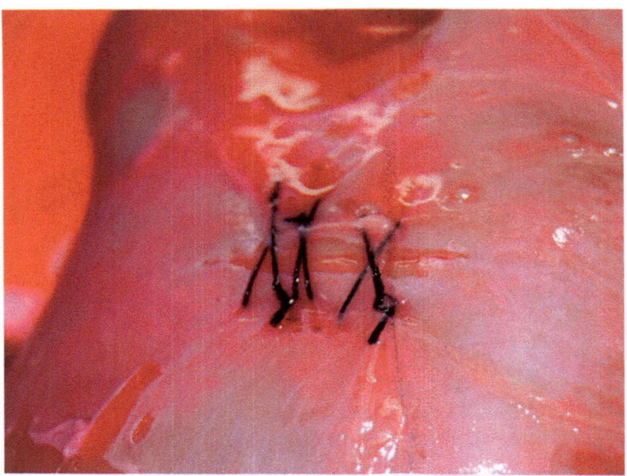

Fig. 4.10 Completion of the task

4.5 Anatomizing the Orange

4.5.1 Objectives

To develop the advanced skills of two-handed maneuvers

4.5.2 Station Setup

Semicircular-shaped simulator
Laparoscopic camera system (Storz)
One pair of laparoscopic scissors
One pair of laparoscopic Maryland forceps

4.5.3 How to Make the Training Model

The material used for practicing is orange.

4.5.4 Description of the Training Procedure (Fig. 4.11)

Step 1: In a box trainer, the orange is peeled with the grasper and the scissors.
Step 2: After peeling, the trainee should clean the fibrous surface segment.
Step 3: The segments are separated.
Step 4: At last, the trainee needs to remove the capsule of each segment.

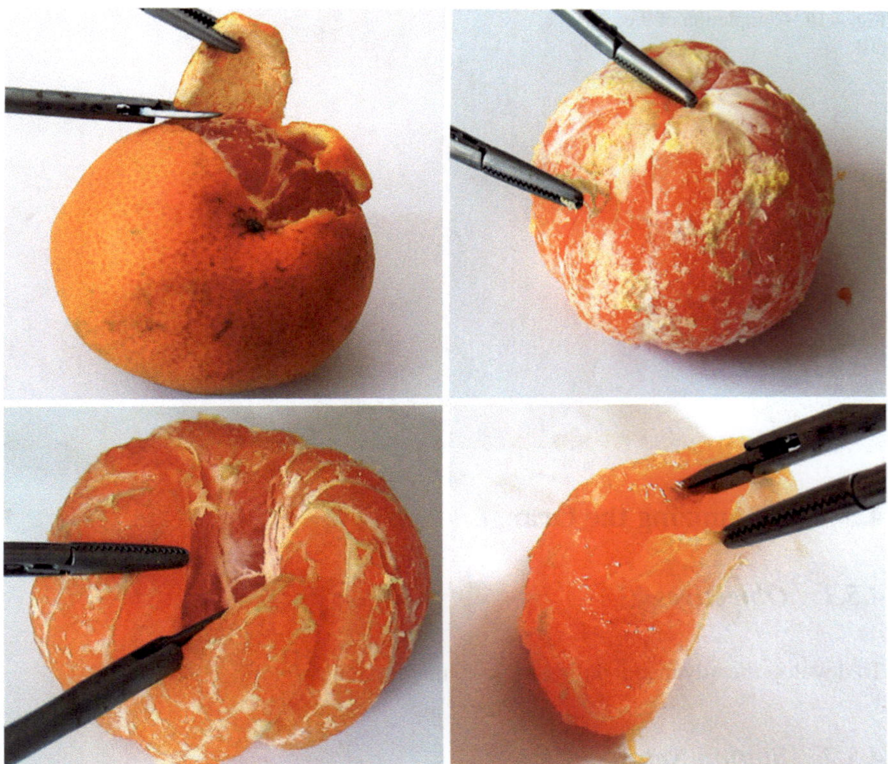

Fig. 4.11 Anatomizing the orange

References

1. Laird A, Stewart GD, Hou S, et al. A novel bovine model for training urological surgeons in laparoscopic radical nephrectomy. J Endourol. 2011;25:1377–83.
2. Abboudi M, Ahmed K, Kirby R, et al. Mentorship programmes for laparoscopic and robotic urology. BJU Int. 2011;107:1869–71.
3. Torricelli FC, Guglielmetti G, Duarte RJ, et al. Laparoscopic skill laboratory in urological surgery: tools and methods for resident training. Int Braz J Urol. 2011;37:108–11. discussion 112.
4. Chung SD, Tai HC, Lai MK, et al. Novel inanimate training model for urethrovesical anastomosis in laparoscopic radical prostatectomy. Asian J Surg. 2010;33:188–92.
5. Autorino R, Haber GP, Stein RJ, et al. Laparoscopic training in urology: critical analysis of current evidence. J Endourol. 2010;24:1377–90.
6. Yang B, Zhang ZS, Xiao L, et al. A novel training model for retroperitoneal laparoscopic dismembered pyeloplasty. J Endourol. 2010;24:1345–9.
7. Yang B, Zeng Q, Yinghao S, et al. A novel training model for laparoscopic partial nephrectomy using porcine kidney. J Endourol. 2009;23:2029–33.
8. Wang H, Yang B, Xu C, et al. New practical course for laparoscopy training: anatomizing the orange. Eur Surg Res. 2009;42:106–8.

Chapter 5
The Laparoscopic Animal Lab Training Module

Ying Hao Sun, Zhenjie Wu, and Bo Yang

Abstract Live animal surgery still represents the best training models compared with other models due to technical limitation, which can provide full capability of encompassing all the aspects of a real surgical experience. In this chapter, tips and tricks for the organization of animal lab are detailed. And guidelines of partial nephrectomy and pyeloplasty are well described.

Keywords Animal lab • Urology • Laparoscopy • Organization • Technique Training

5.1 Introduction

Following the rapid development of computer technology, nowadays special softwares allow virtual reality (VR) trainers to simulate many kinds of surgical procedures by assessing the performance in terms of completion time, errors, and economy of motion and cautery [1]. This has been proposed as the future of laparoscopic surgical training.

However, up to now, due to technical limitations, the VR trainer cannot very realistically mimic a surgical situation. Because of this, live animal surgery still represents the best training models, offering a level of fidelity unmatched by any other form of simulation model [2, 3].

Y.H. Sun, M.D. (✉) • Z. Wu, M.D. • B. Yang, M.D.
Department of Urology, Changhai Hospital,
168 Changhai Road, Shanghai 200433, China
e-mail: sunyh@medmail.com.cn

Y.H. Sun et al. (eds.), *The Training Courses of Urological Laparoscopy*,
DOI 10.1007/978-1-4471-2723-9_5,

When trainees enter an animal lab, facing the operating room environment, they will likely feel a realistic excitement and pressure because of possible complications that can occur during this kind of training. Their surgical skills and judgment will be fully displayed and assessed [4, 5].

No other training simulator can provide such full capability of encompassing all the aspects of a real surgical experience. It is for this reason that the American College of Surgeons "believes that now and in the foreseeable future it is not possible to completely replace the use of animals and that the study of whole living organisms, tissues, and cells is an indispensable element of biomedical research, education, and teaching" and "supports the use and humane care and treatment of laboratory animals in research, education, teaching, and product safety testing in accordance with applicable local, state, and federal animal welfare laws" [6].

However, for the novices, it is not easy to gain the opportunity to practice in the animal lab due to the high cost and the ethical issue, which is not the case for dry lab training. Therefore, how to make a good use of the live animal model represents a valuable topic [7].

5.2 Animal Lab Organization: Tips and Tricks

Live animal surgery is a teamwork. It is necessary to have a preparatory meeting among all team members the night before the animal lab day. The second import thing is that the trainees should have previous experience in the dry lab. If not, they have to spend half a day to do an intensive training before the animal lab. The last thing is that a visual support with videos of animal surgical procedures should be made available to every trainee. The material should include positioning of the animal, principles of animal anatomy, and a step-by-step procedure guideline. The trainee can study these videos and understand these basic steps and key points before having access to the live animal surgery.

Regarding the operation, we recommend to focus on bilateral partial nephrectomy and pyeloplasty. For the simple nephrectomy, it is relatively easy because of the lack of perirenal fat in the porcine model. Of course, the trainee should practice to clip and divide the renal vessels at the end of animal lab.

Last, video recording of the training session can be a desirable gift for the participating trainee.

5.3 Animal Lab: Guidelines

5.3.1 Learning Objectives

1. To understand the basic surgical steps of transperitoneal partial nephrectomy and pyeloplasty

2. To gain skills in meticulous dissection and reconstructive techniques
3. To practice in surgical judgment during a live surgery

5.3.2 Laparoscopic Instruments

Veress needles (1), 5-mm (2) and 10-mm trocars (3), J-Hook electrode (1), Maryland dissector forceps (1), bowel graspers (1), monopolar scissors (1), suction device (1) and needle drivers (2). Satinsky vascular clamp (1) or bulldogs (2)
Vicryl 4-0, 2-0 and 0 sutures, 5-mm Hem-o-lok clips (10) and clip applier (1)

5.3.3 Animal Position and Access Placement

The operating room configuration is showed in the Fig. 5.1. The swine is initially positioned supine for IV access, induction of general anesthesia, and endotracheal intubation (Fig. 5.2). After the orogastric tube is placed, it can be changed to the flank position. For a better exposure, it is important to insert the roll pad under the porcine back.

Relevant bony landmarks and lateral border of the rectus muscle should be marked, including the costal margin, the tip of 12th rib, and the anterior/superior iliac spine. The porcine kidney should be close to the level of 12th rib.

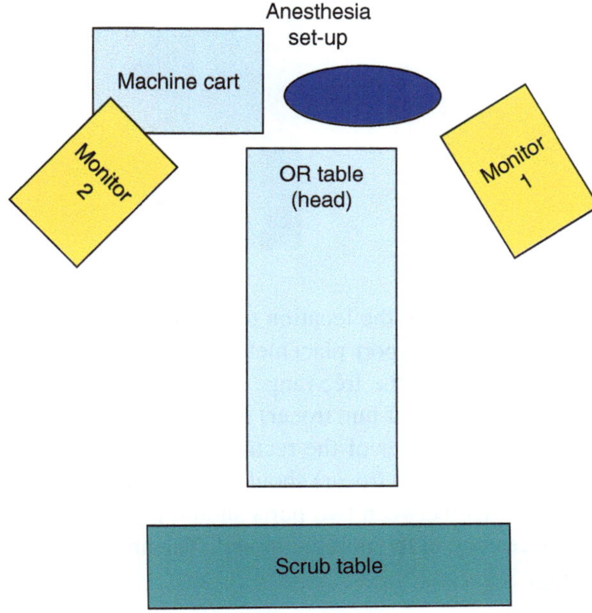

Fig. 5.1 The setup of animal lab

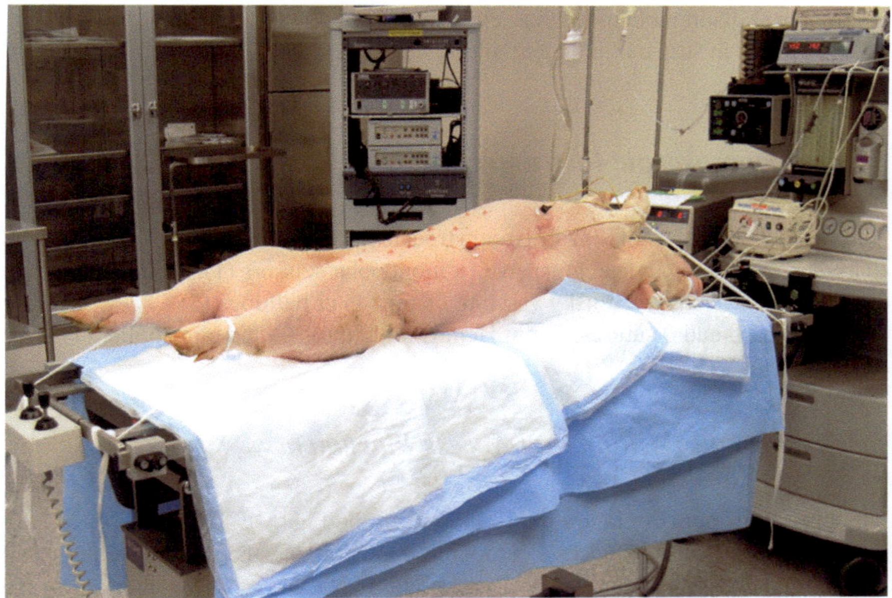

Fig. 5.2 Supine position before induction of general anesthesia

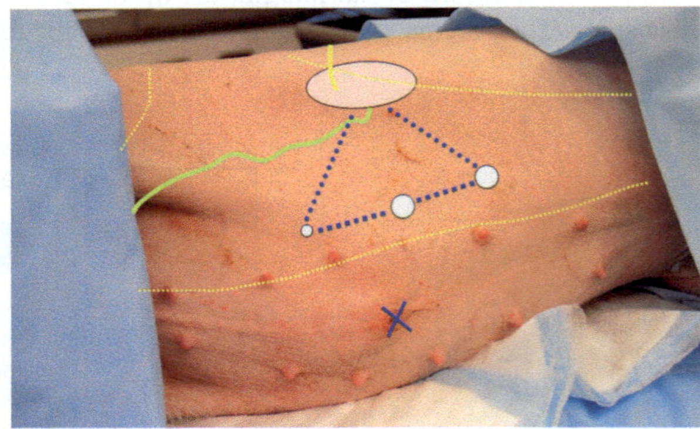

Fig. 5.3 The anticipated location of ports for kidney surgery

How to choose the location of trocars is one of the key points for a successful animal lab. Good port placement can optimize the visualization of the operative field and provide the free range of motion (instruments triangulation). Generally, the camera port (10-mm trocar) should be placed at the level of 12th rib and closed to the lateral border of the rectus muscle. The lower port (5-mm trocar) and the upper port (12-mm trocar) should be placed at the same line with the camera port. The distance between two ports should be kept at least 10 cm. Liver retraction is not necessary in the porcine model. The anticipated location of ports are showed in Fig. 5.3.

5.4 Step-by-Step Technique of Living Animal Lab

5.4.1 Establishment of Pneumoperitoneum

If a Veress needle technique is chosen, it should be known that this can be more difficult than an actual human being. Firstly, a 12-mm incision is made in the anticipated location of camera port (Fig. 5.4). Then, the subcutaneous tissue and muscle layer should be dissected bluntly with the Kelly clamp (Fig. 5.5). With two Allis clamp grasping the skin and subcutaneous tissue, the Veress needle is passed through the peritoneum (Fig. 5.6).

After the aspiration/irrigation test and the hanging drop test, insufflation is started (Fig. 5.7). The trainee should pay close attention to the abdominal shape and the intra-abdominal pressure. If irregular abdominal dilation or rapid increasing pressure is noted, the Veress needle might not have passed through the peritoneum. In this

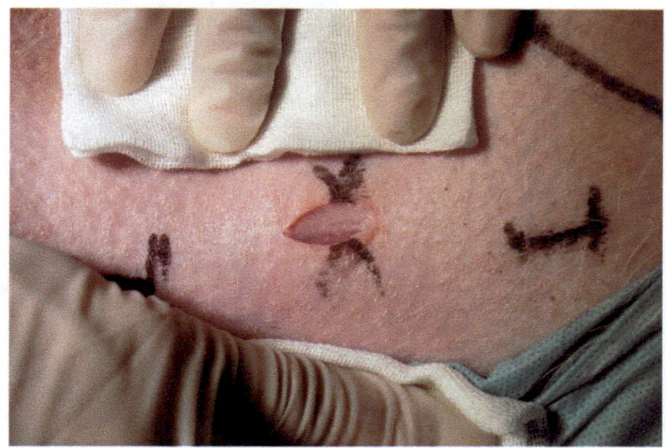

Fig. 5.4 To make the first incision at the camera position

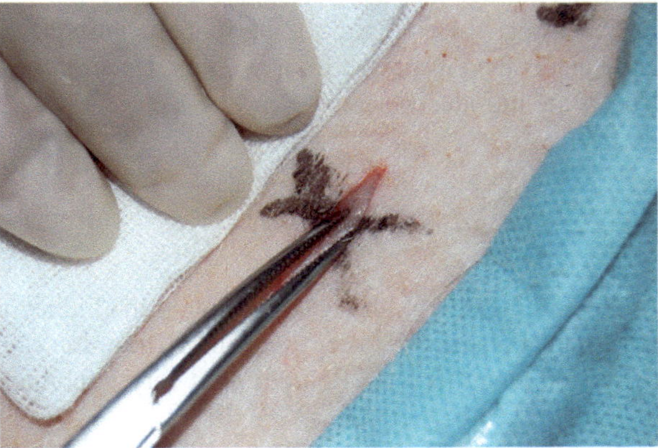

Fig. 5.5 To bluntly dissect the muscle layer with the Kelly clamp

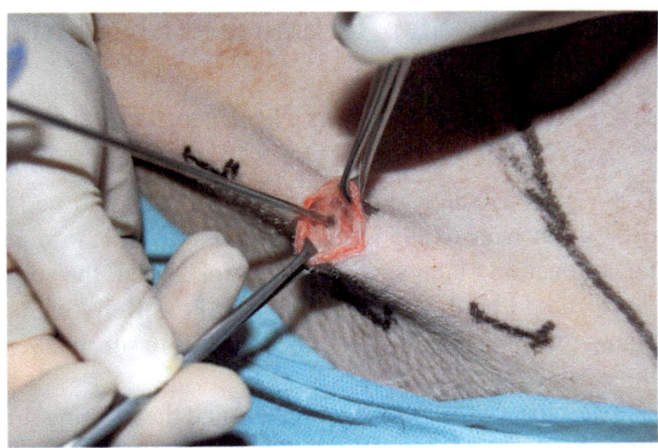

Fig. 5.6 To place the Veress needle

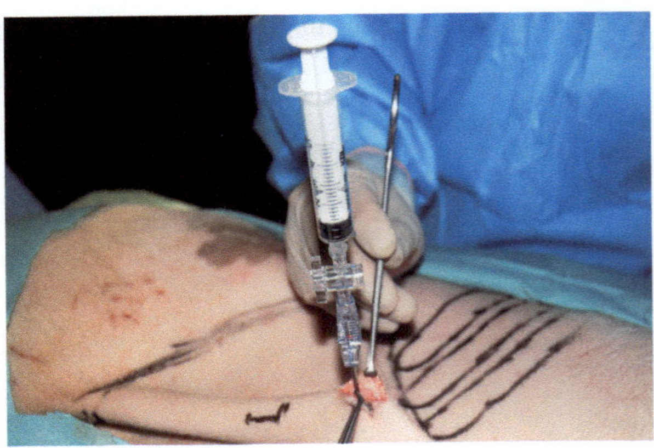

Fig. 5.7 The aspiration/irrigation test

case, one should remove it and do the maneuver again. If it fails more than twice, the open access technique should be adopted, and it can be done more easily.

Once pneumoperitoneum pressure is reached at the15 mmHg, the 10-mm trocar is passed through the same incision (Fig. 5.8). After warming the camera and cleaning the trocar valve (Fig. 5.9), the scope is introduced through the trocar, and the abdomen is then inspected for any injury. Under direct vision, the second and third trocars are introduced safely.

5.4.2 Partial Nephrectomy

In the porcine model, the fat surrounding the kidney is much less than in human. Anatomical planes are easier to identify. The colon can be mobilized medially with dissection along its lateral border. It is very important to maintain clear anatomic

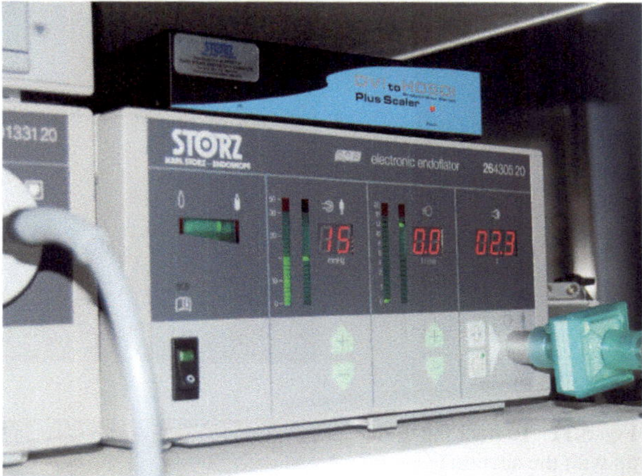

Fig. 5.8 The 15 mmHg pneumoperitoneum pressure before introducing the camera trocar

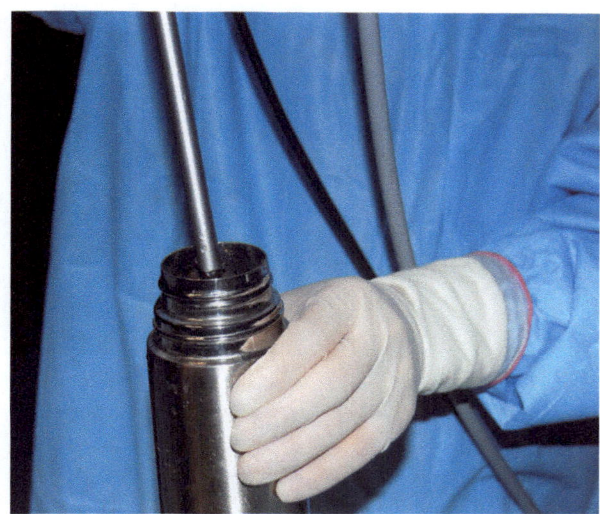

Fig. 5.9 To warm the camera with hot water

plane. The colon should be pushed down by the bowel grasper to get enough tension. Note that an effective countertraction provides the necessary tension that is a key point during laparoscopic dissection. The left hand should grasp or push the right tissue at the right time to provide good exposure and tension for right hand. The renal hilum will be exposed after enough colon mobilization (Fig. 5.10).

At the level of the lower pole of the kidney, the ureter can be easily found. Then, the ureter can be lift by using the left hand with suction or bowel grasper. It is advisable not to divide it so that further dissection of renal hilum will be much easier (Fig. 5.11). Following the ureter and the surface of the psoas muscle, tissues between the kidney and great vessels can be dissected towards the renal hilum (Fig. 5.12).

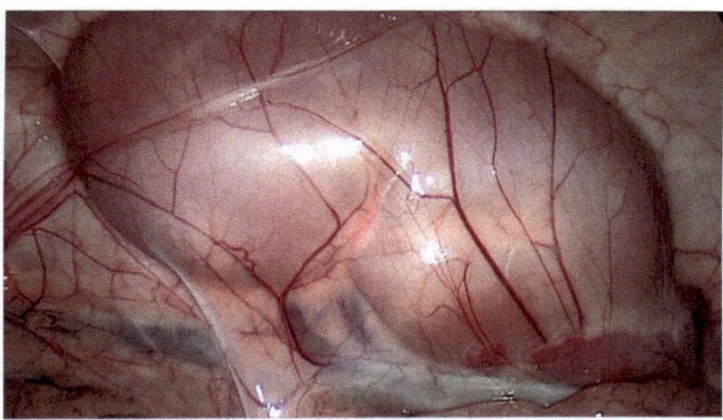

Fig. 5.10 The right kidney

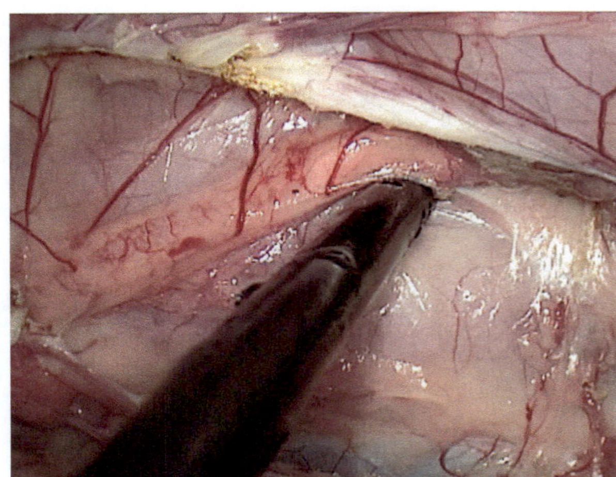

Fig. 5.11 To tract the ureter up with the suction

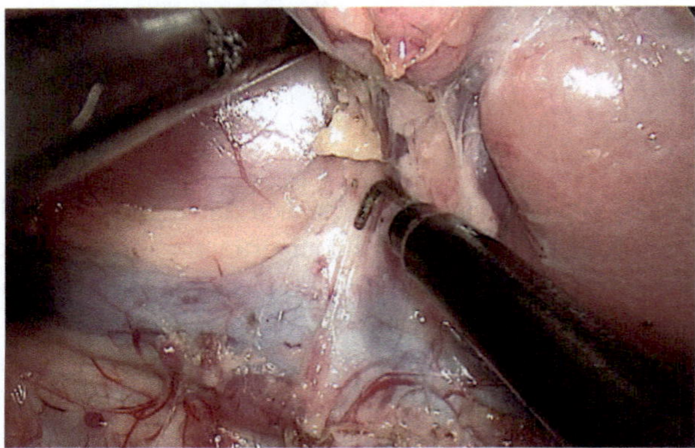

Fig. 5.12 The renal hilum

By gently pushing up the kidney by the left hand's suction, the renal hilum is brought under tension. Note that keeping this tension is very important for a successful dissection of the vessels. The superficial fascia of the renal vein can be removed by using the hook. Another tip at this point is to expose first in order to

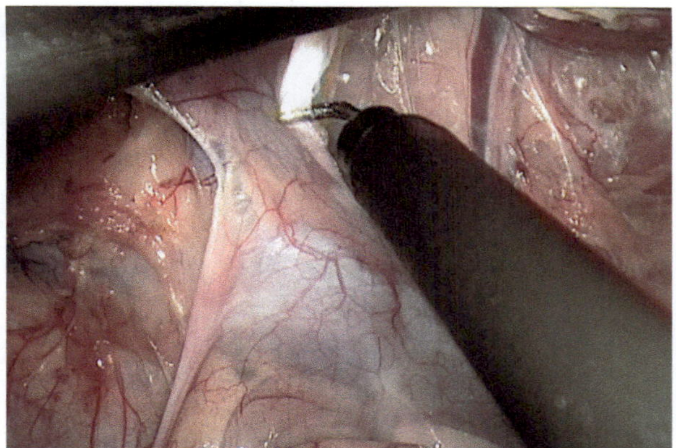

Fig. 5.13 To free the renal vein

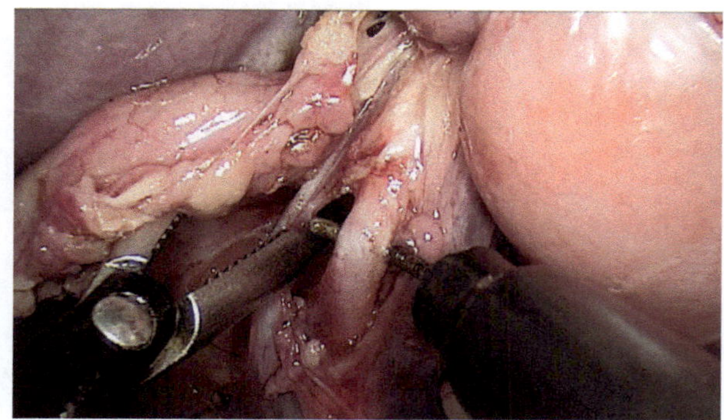

Fig. 5.14 To dissect the renal artery

protect the structure you are dissecting. According to this principle, the more the renal vein is freed, the safer its management becomes (Fig. 5.13). This step of the procedure is a very valuable exercise for the trainee to get confidence with hook manipulation.

The renal artery is always lying either right behind or slightly superior to the renal vein. After the renal vein is dissected, we can insert the suction or Maryland dissector forceps to the space between the renal vein and artery and push the renal vein aside gently (Fig. 5.14). This is a useful tip to expose the renal artery. Then, the renal artery can be easily freed.

The Gerota's fascia overlying the anticipated area should be removed. For the novice, the anterior interpolar region of the kidney is a more suitable location to perform the "tumor resection."

Please check if everything is ready before the hilum is clamped, including the suture with clip, the bulldogs, or the Satinsky clamp (Fig. 5.15). The length of the suture has to be 7–10 cm, and the "sliding clip" knotless technique is recommended to close the kidney.

After the hilum is clamped, the "tumor" should be excised with cold scissors in a bloodless operative field (Fig. 5.16). If one needs to get a better angle to excise the "tumor," an additional trocar can be added as needed.

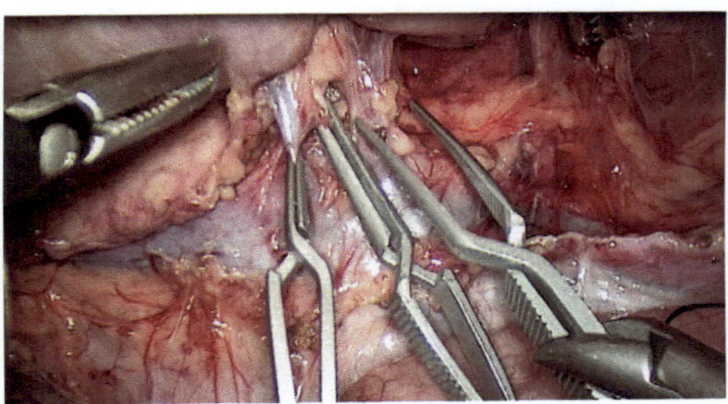

Fig. 5.15 To clamp the renal artery and vein with bulldogs

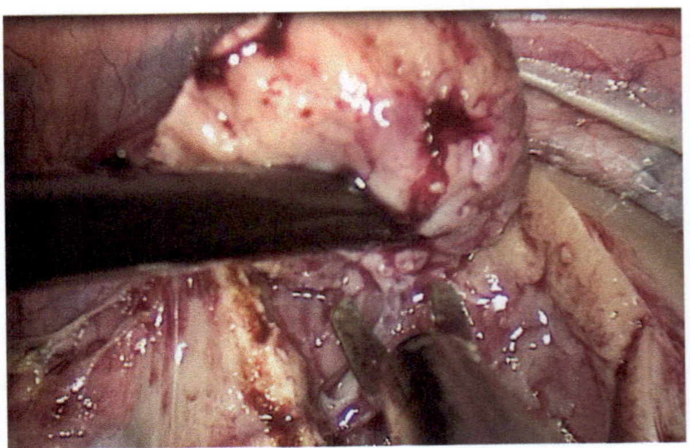

Fig. 5.16 To excise the "tumor" with scissors

Renal reconstruction should include two parts: the deep layer (pelvicalyceal closure) and the parenchymal layer. For the deep layer, a running suture method can be used with a 2-0 Vicryl on CT-1 needle. For the parenchymal layer, a "U-shaped" continuous suture method can be used with a 0 Vicryl on CTX needle anchored by the mental clips (Fig. 5.17). After removing the clamp, in the actively bleeding wound, further parenchymal sutures can be placed with the 0 Vicryl to achieve complete hemostasis (Fig. 5.18).

5.4.3 Pyeloplasty

In the normal porcine model, it is very rare to have a dilated pelvis. Thus, this procedure in this case is in fact a ureteroureterostomy. For the novice surgeon, this can be a challenging task. So, we recommend that this procedure should be carried out after bilateral partial nephrectomy.

At the level of the lower pole of the kidney, ureter can be identified and dissected up and down at least 2 cm (Fig. 5.19).

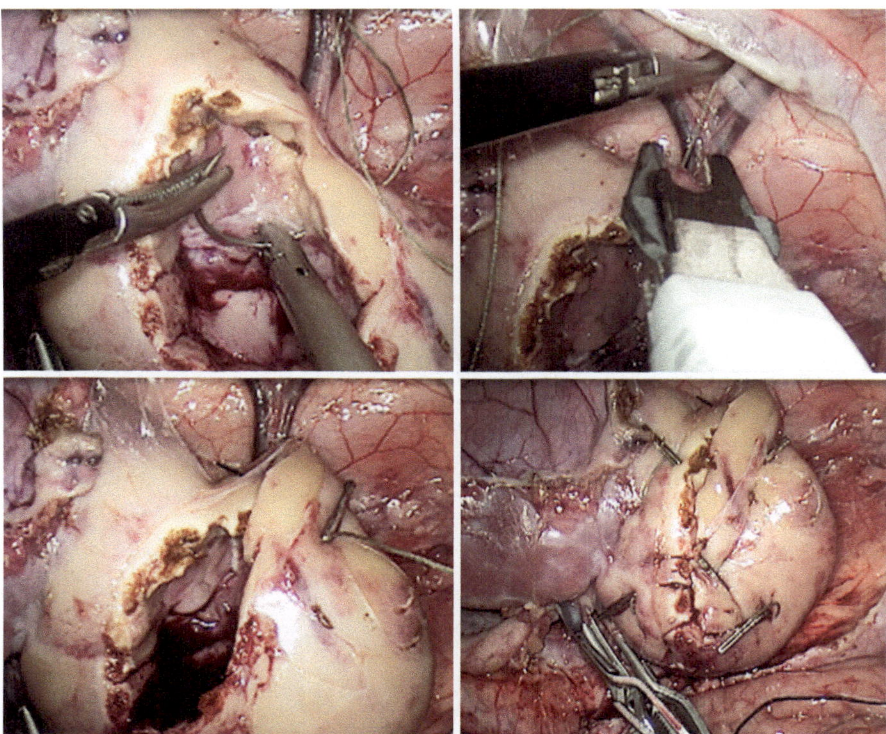

Fig. 5.17 Knotless parenchymal renorrhaphy with mental clip

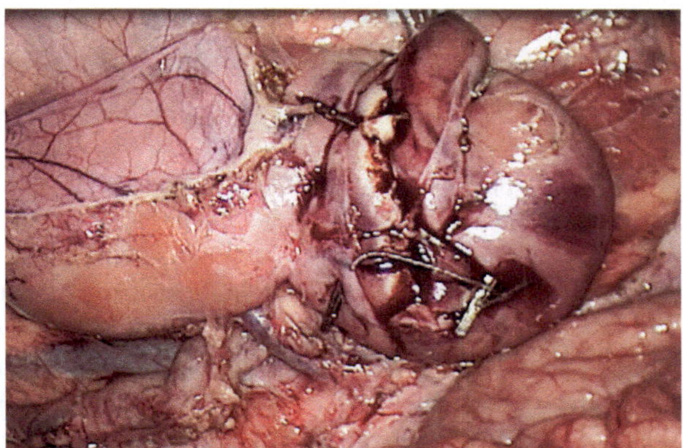

Fig. 5.18 To remove bulldogs

The ureter is cut and spatulation is performed for both ureteral segments at 180 degrees apart over 1 cm (Fig. 5.20). At this point, for novice, it may be difficult to find the ureteral lumen and insert one blade of scissors' tip into it because of the lack of enough stability. To overcome this issue, a tip can be that before excision, the

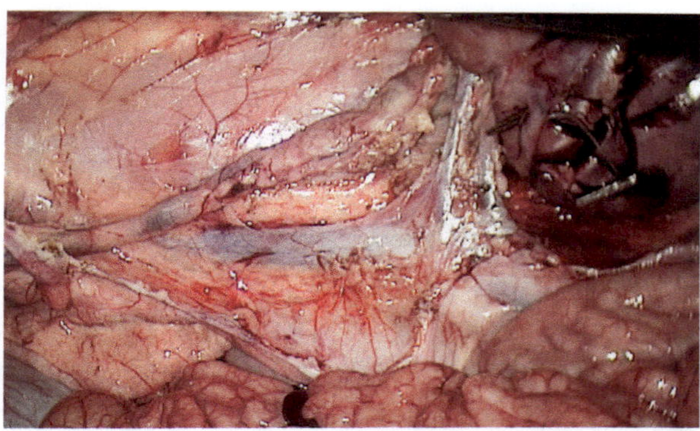

Fig. 5.19 To dissect 4-cm ureter for pyeloplasty

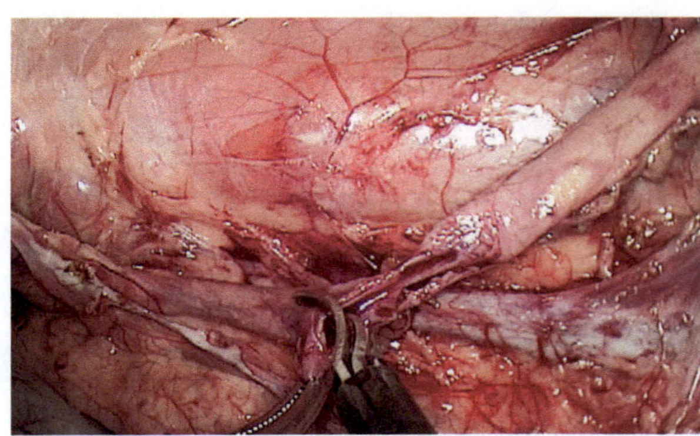

Fig. 5.20 To spatulate the ureter up and down

ureter can be fixed on the surface of the psoas muscle by placing a stay suture. Then, the ureter can be cut incompletely and spatulated (Fig. 5.21).

A 4-0 Vicryl suture (10 cm) is passed through the edge of the other ureteral segment from outside to inside. Then it is passed through the ureteral wall at the "V-shaped" apex from inside to outside and tied (Fig. 5.22). The same procedure is done on the opposite side. The tip in this case is to keep the end of the suture at least 3–4 cm length so that it can be fixed on the psoas muscle fascia with clips (Fig. 5.23).

The anastomosis of the anterior wall can then be completed by running these two sutures continuously or in an interrupted fashion. Generally, three stitches are enough. Sometimes the novice falls into trouble when trying to find the ureteral edge. The tip here is to use the needle tip to lift up the tissue around the ureter edge, then hold the edge by using a Maryland dissector forceps (Fig. 5.24).

When the anterior wall is done, the ureter is to be rotated by 180 degrees and two ends of the suture fixed on the psoas muscle fascia. Then the posterior wall of the ureter will be exposed very nicely. The same thing can be done on the opposite side (Fig. 5.25).

If possible, one can practice in the placement of a double J stent before completion of the anastomotic closure. This can be another challenging surgical task.

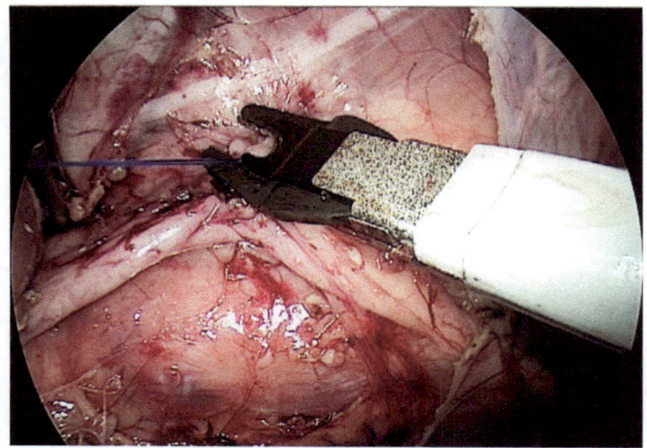

Fig. 5.21 To fix the ureter on the muscle surface

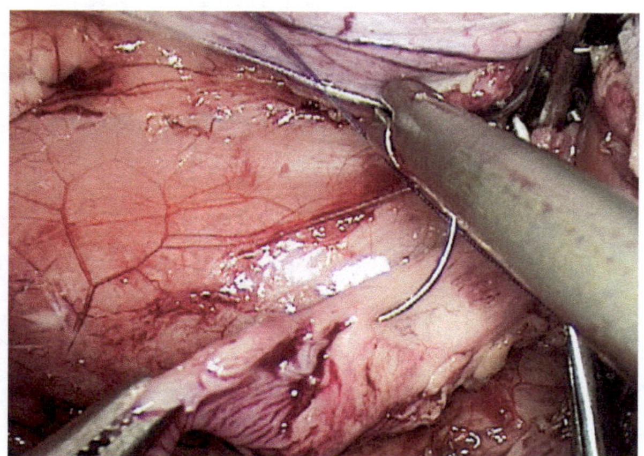

Fig. 5.22 The first suture at the "V-shaped" apex of the ureter

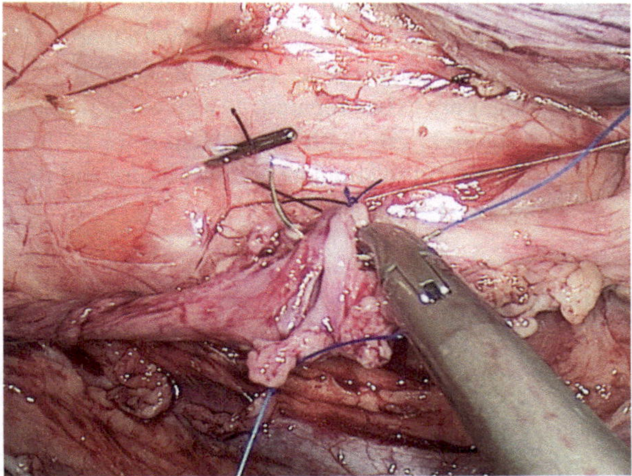

Fig. 5.23 To fix the ureter on the psoas muscle during the anastomosis of the anterior wall

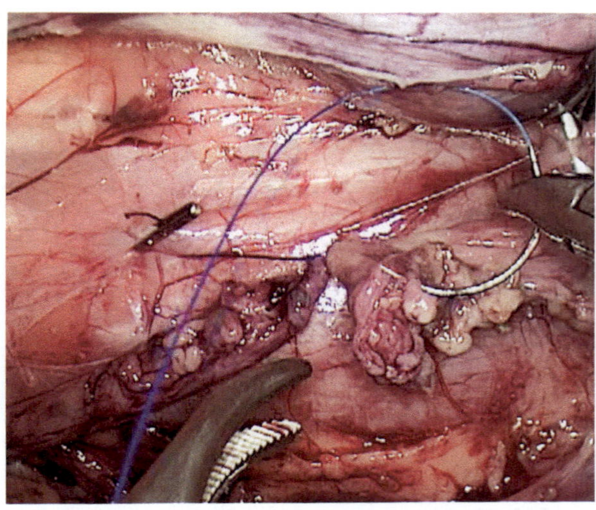

Fig. 5.24 To lift the ureter edge with needle tip

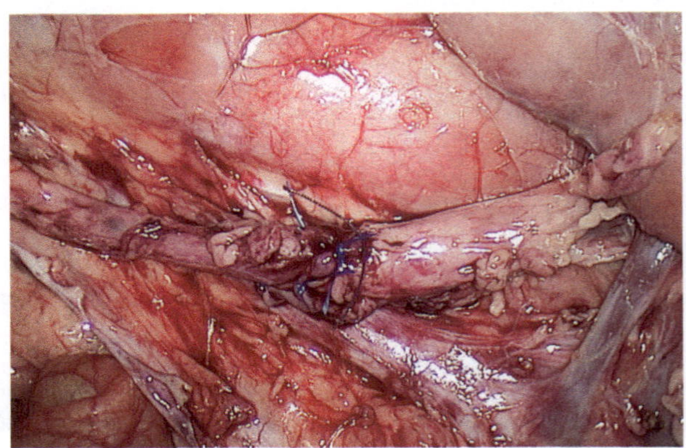

Fig. 5.25 To complete the anastomosis of the posterior wall

When all of the procedures are completed and the porcine is still live, there is still a good opportunity to further test its own laparoscopic skills. How to control an intraoperative major bleeding can be a valuable challenge for the novice. Some gauze sponges are to be prepared, as well as suction, needle driver, additional trocar, and a 2-0 suture (7 cm) with 5-mm Hem-o-lok at the end. Then, the vena cava can be intentionally cut to simulate a vessel injury and its laparoscopic management.

References

1. Ramirez-Backhaus M, Hellawell G, Melo M, et al. Teaching laparoscopy to residents: how can we select good candidates? Curr Urol Rep. 2009;10:106–11.
2. Fearn SJ, Burke K, Hartley DE, et al. A laparoscopic access technique for endovascular procedures: surgeon training in an animal model. J Endovasc Ther. 2006;13:350–6.

3. Kirlum HJ, Heinrich M, Tillo N, et al. Advanced paediatric laparoscopic surgery: repetitive training in a rabbit model provides superior skills for live operations. Eur J Pediatr Surg. 2005;15:149–52.
4. Mori T, Hatano N, Maruyama S, et al. Significance of "hands-on training" in laparoscopic surgery. Surg Endosc. 1998;12:256–60.
5. Böhm B, Milsom JW. Animal models as educational tools in laparoscopic colorectal surgery. Surg Endosc. 1994;8:707–13.
6. Byrne P. Teaching laparoscopic surgery. Practice on live animals is illegal. BMJ. 1994;308:1435.
7. Wolfe BM, Szabo Z, Moran ME, et al. Training for minimally invasive surgery. Need for surgical skills. Surg Endosc. 1993;7:93–5.

Chapter 6
The Laparoendoscopic Single-Site Surgery (LESS) Training Module

Ying Hao Sun, Bo Yang, Huiqing Wang, Liang Xiao, and Zhenjie Wu

Abstract The development of laparoendoscopic single-site surgery (LESS) represents the future step forward in the field of minimally invasive surgery compared with traditional laparoscopy. In this chapter, different kinds of access devices and instruments for LESS are documented. Considering LESS is technically more challenging than standard laparoscopy, three specialized training courses are designed to train LESS basic skills which is also well described in this chapter. Besides, authors represent their opinions about the challenges of LESS; robotic LESS is also briefly introduced.

Keywords Laparoendoscopic single-site surgery • Learning curve • Basic skill • Training • Model

6.1 Current Status of Laparoendoscopic Single-Site Surgery (LESS) in Urology

6.1.1 Introduction

Beginning in the early 1990s, laparoscopy has evolved to become the standard technique for many urological procedures [1, 2]. Even for more difficult and advanced procedures, such as partial nephrectomy and radical prostatectomy, laparoscopy has become an option in hands of skilled surgeons [3–5].

Y.H. Sun, M.D. (✉) • B. Yang, M.D. • H. Wang, M.D. • L. Xiao, M.E. • Z. Wu, M.D.
Department of Urology, Changhai Hospital,
168 Changhai Road, Shanghai 200433, China
e-mail: sunyh@medmail.com.cn

Y.H. Sun et al. (eds.), *The Training Courses of Urological Laparoscopy*,
DOI 10.1007/978-1-4471-2723-9_6, © Springer-Verlag London 2012

A further step forward in the field of minimally invasive surgery has been more recently represented by the development of laparoendoscopic single-site surgery (LESS). This technique has been introduced with the aim of minimizing surgery-related morbidity and optimizing the cosmetic outcome toward a virtually “scar-less” surgery. This newly developed surgical technique challenges the main principles of conventional multiport laparoscopy.

LESS appendectomy was first described in 1992 [6], whereas the first LESS cholecystectomy was reported in 1997 [7]. In urology, the first LESS cases, consisting of simple nephrectomy, were reported by Rane et al. in 2007 [8]. Since then, a broad spectrum of urologic procedures has been reported and shown to be feasible. In 2009, the first two large (100 cases) series on LESS in urology were reported [9, 10]. Despite some controversial issues, with LESS, a new era has just begun in the field of operative urology [11]

6.1.2 Less Access

In LESS, the incision always hides inside the umbilicus in order to avoid a visible surgical “scar.” A challenging and critical aspect of LESS is to establish a transumbilicus access with a single small incision [12].

Many companies have developed innovative multichannel ports, and some surgeons have reported the use of homemade access devices for LESS [13].

The following access devices and techniques have been described:

6.1.2.1 Multiple Low-Profile Trocars Through the Same Incision (Fig. 6.1)

A skin incision around the umbilicus ring is made, and three low-profile 5-mm trocars are inserted. The major drawback of this method is represented by the crowding of these trocars which are too close.

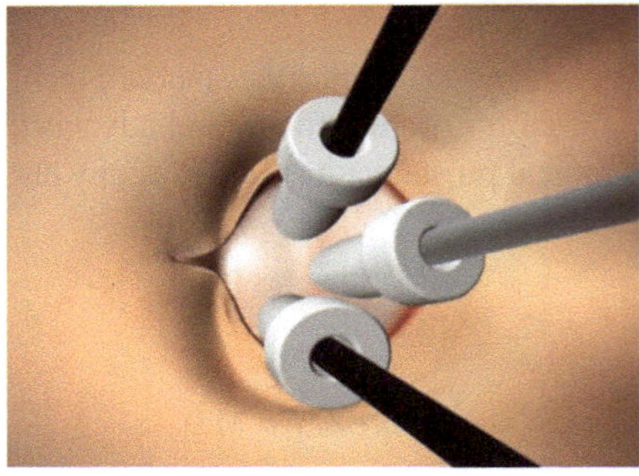

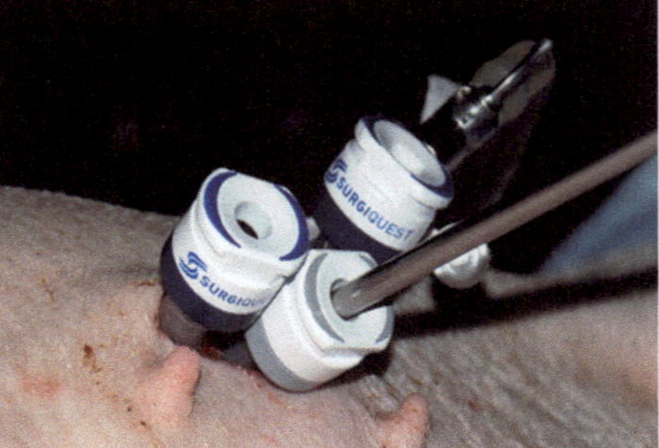

Fig. 6.1 Multiple small trocars in a line

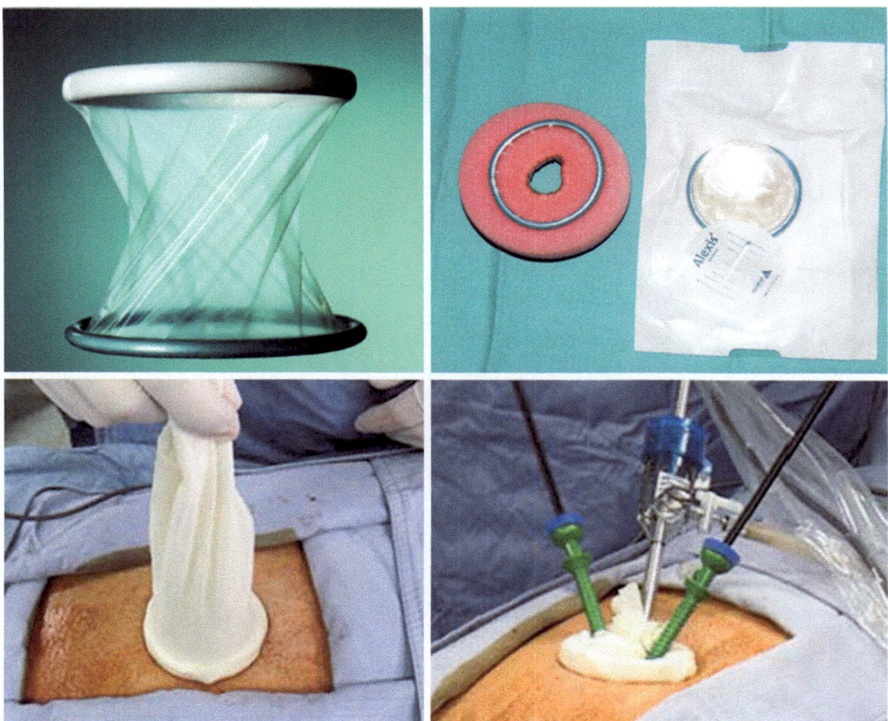

Fig. 6.2 Homemade access by the surgical glove

6.1.2.2 **Homemade Access Device** (Fig. 6.2)

An Alexis wound retractor is introduced in position through the umbilical incision with the bottom ring inside the abdomen. A sterile surgical glove is attached to the external ring and in this way secured to the abdominal wall. Standard laparoscopic trocar is then inserted through the glove and fixed.

6.1.2.3 **TriPort™ (Olympus)** (Fig. 6.3)

This is a common multichannel port with three access sites (one 12 mm, two 5 mm) and two valves for insufflations and smoke evacuation. It is easy to place with the aid of an introducer, and it is advantageous for obese patients with a thick abdominal wall because of the adjustable length of the port sleeve.

6.1.2.4 **SILS™ Port (Covidien)** (Fig. 6.4)

The SILS port has the shape of the wine cork with three holes. It is made of a special foamy material with an excellent deformability. The surgeon can choose different

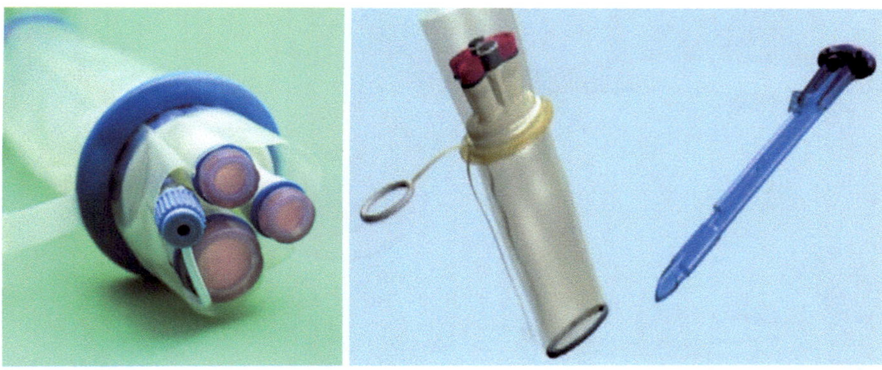

Fig. 6.3 TriPort access device

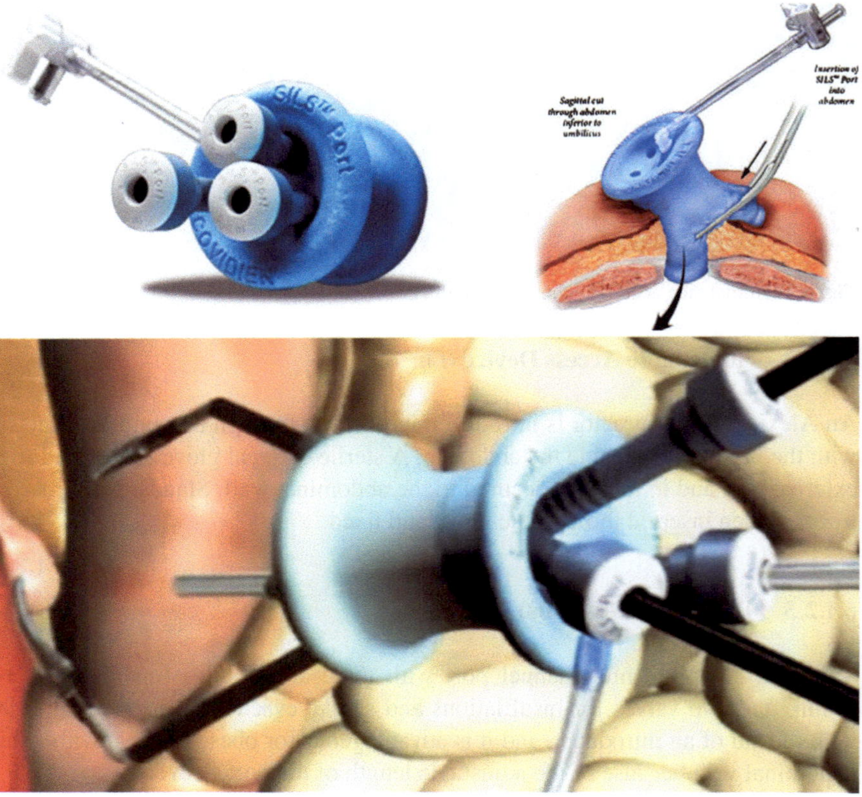

Fig. 6.4 SILS access device

combination of the trocars (three 5 mm or two 12 mm, and one 5 mm) according to the procedure. It is more challenging to place than the TriPort, especially for obese patients.

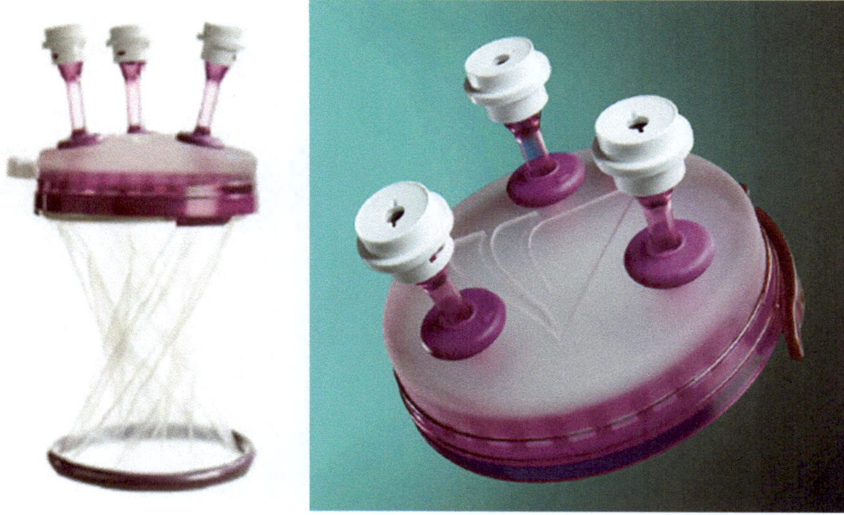

Fig. 6.5 GelPOINT access device

6.1.2.5 GelPOINT™ (Applied Medical) (Fig. 6.5)

This multichannel system is developed from the hand-assisted laparoscopy device GelPort. The wound retractor can accommodate 1.5-cm to 7-cm incisions and varied abdominal wall thickness for wide spectrum of procedures. It allows extracorporeal anastomosis and large specimen retrieval, such as those of radical nephrectomy and cystectomy.

6.1.2.6 X-CONE™ and ENDOCONE™ (Karl Storz) (Figs. 6.6 and 6.7)

They are two kinds of reusable metallic multichannel port, which have valves for multiple telescope and instrument access. The working channels of X-CONE permit the introduction of instruments up to 12.5 mm in size (clip applicator, stapler, etc.).

6.1.2.7 Single Site Laparoscopy Access System (Ethicon Endo-Surgery) (Fig. 6.8)

This port is somewhat similar to the TriPort systems. There are two available sizes of the retractor (2 cm, 4 cm) for the patients with variety of abdominal wall thickness. With the insertion tool, it is easy to place the retractor, and the integrated seal system does not require trocar use, eliminating possible interference between

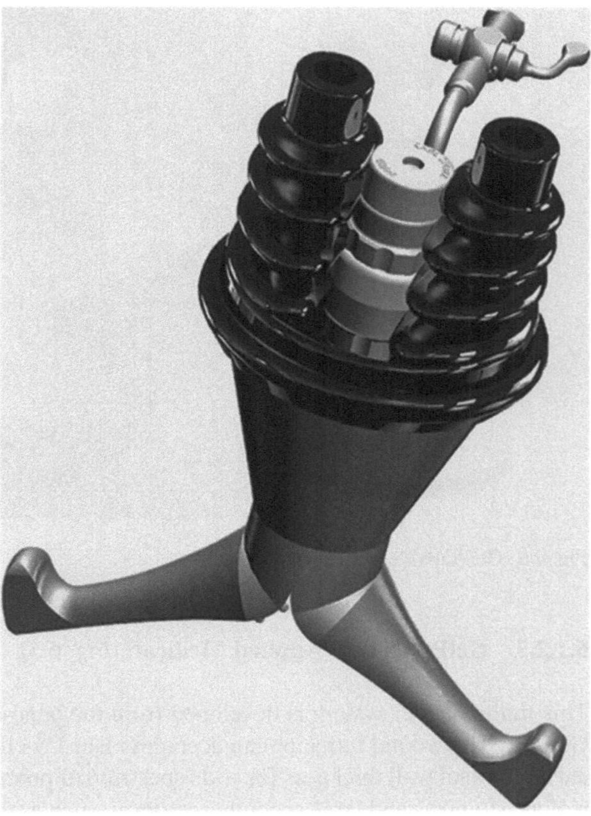

Fig. 6.6 X-CONE access device

trocars. Removable seal cap makes it easy to extract large specimens without removing the device.

6.1.2.8 AirSeal™ (SurgiQuest) (Fig. 6.9)

Without a valve or a gasket, AirSeal maintains pneumoperitoneum by creating an air vortex. Any combination of multiple instruments can be used from the one large opening in the trocar.

6.1.3 Laparoscopic Instruments for Less

Triangulation represents a paradigm for conventional laparoscopy surgery as it provides a comfortable and ergonomic movement of the instruments. And this is critical, for example, when dissecting along anatomical planes and retracting tissue to

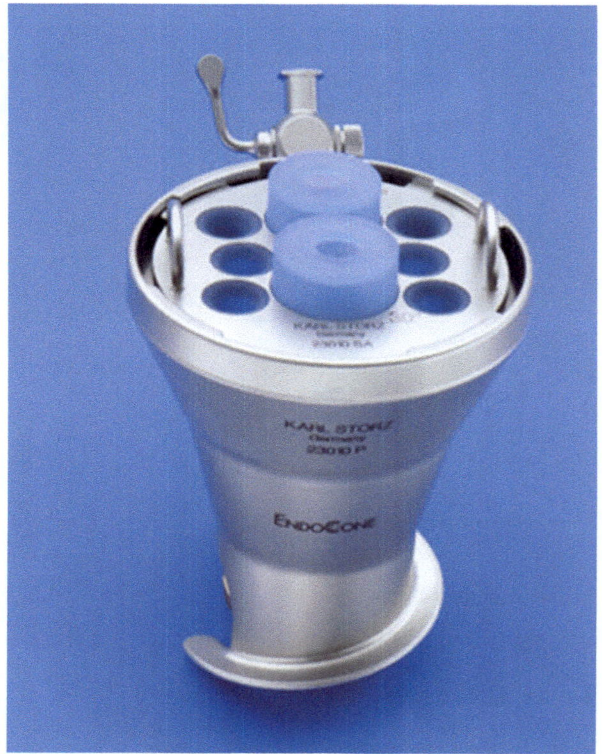

Fig. 6.7 ENDOCONE access device

expose the surgical field. However, in LESS, instruments are placed parallel (chopstick phenomenon) so that triangulation becomes not possible with the use of traditional laparoscopic instruments (Fig. 6.10).

The development of novel flexible/articulating instruments for LESS has allowed to address this key challenge of LESS. Many of these purpose-built instruments have been designed to restore triangulation, also using the crossing method (Fig. 6.11).

For more complex reconstructive surgery, the additional use of 2-mm instrument can be very helpful with minimal additional trauma (Fig. 6.12).

6.1.3.1 Real Hand™ High Dexterity Instruments (Novare Surgical Systems, Cupertino, USA) (Fig. 6.13)

Based on the EndoLink mechanism, they are full range of motion handheld laparoscopic instruments without the additional hardware. When the surgeon's hand moves in one direction, the instrument tip exactly follows. It is helpful to achieve triangulation through a single incision.

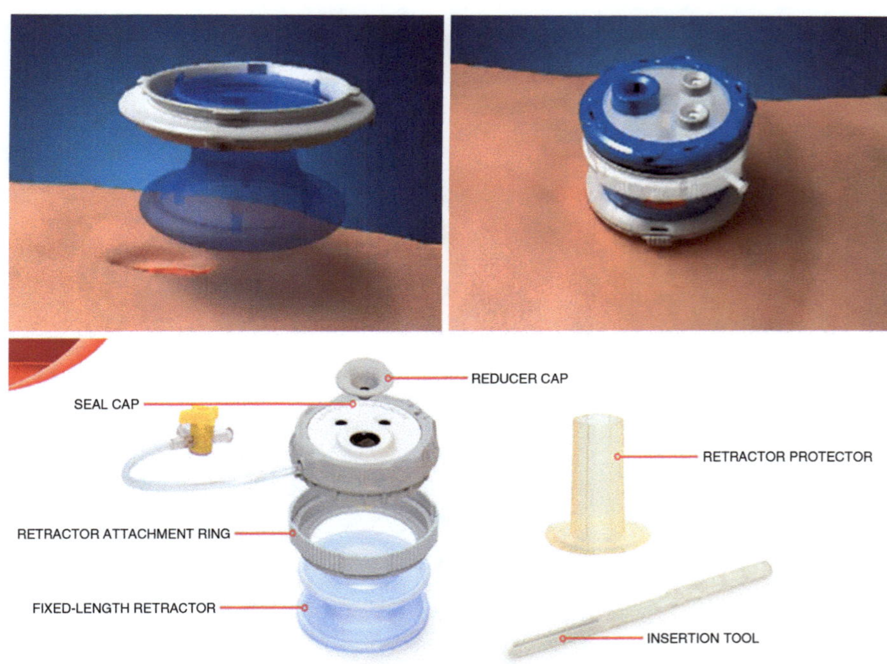

Fig. 6.8 Multichannel access device (Ethicon)

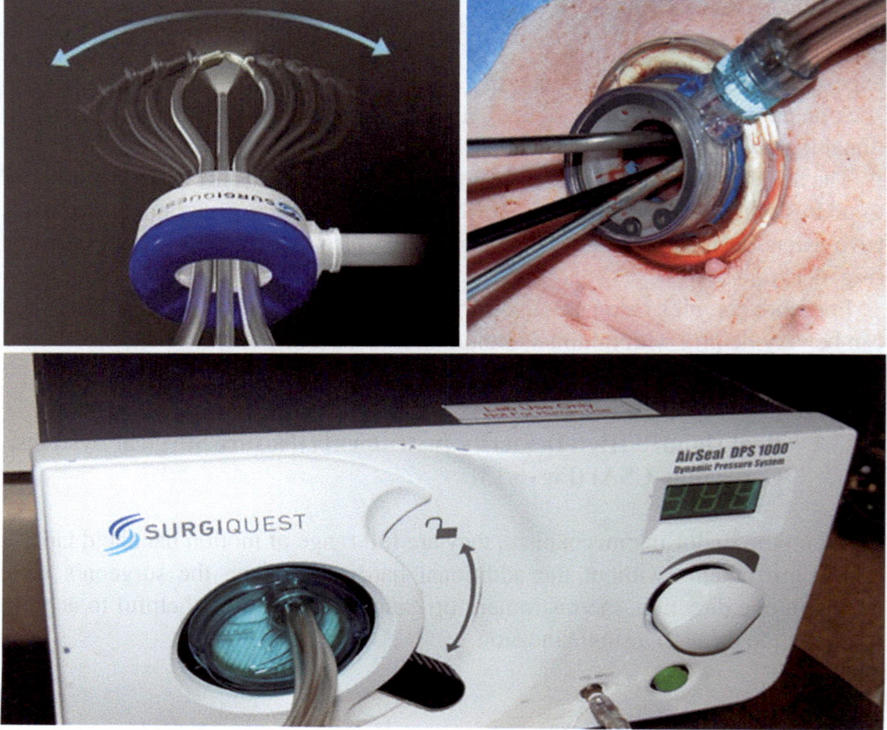

Fig. 6.9 AirSeal system

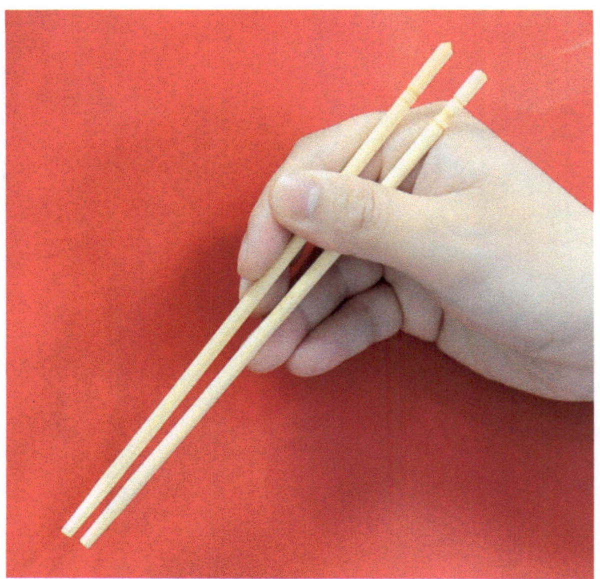

Fig. 6.10 Chopstick phenomenon in LESS

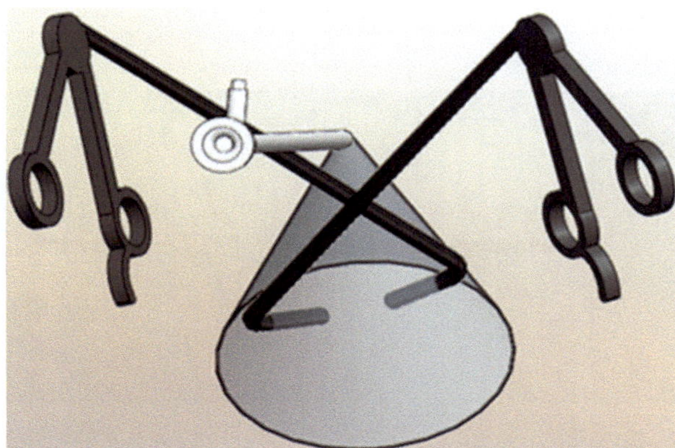

Fig. 6.11 The crossing method of flexible instrument

6.1.3.2 Autonomy Laparo-Angle™ Instruments (Cambridge Endoscopic Devices, Framingham, USA) (Fig. 6.14)

They have seven degrees of freedom, and the tip can rotate 360° around its axis for precise positioning. An important feature is the locking function at any angle. Surgeon's fatigue is minimized and strength of the instruments improved.

6.1.3.3 SILS™ Stitch Articulating Endoscopic Suturing Device (Covidien) (Fig. 6.15)

This is a novel Endo Stitch laparoscopic instrument with distal shaft articulation, needle jaw tip rotation, and additional shaft length. The articulating features of the

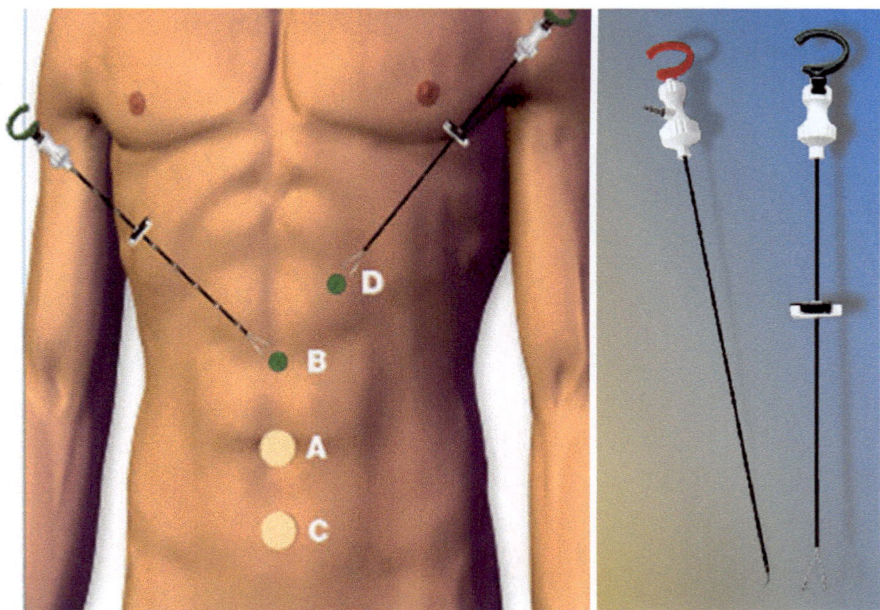

Fig. 6.12 2-mm instrument for additional port

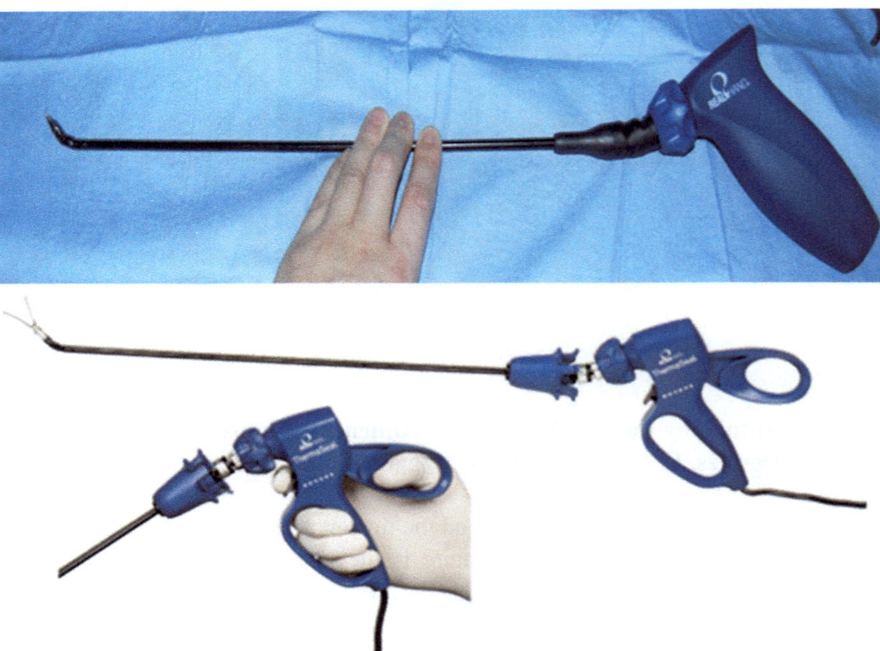

Fig. 6.13 Real Hand™ High Dexterity instruments

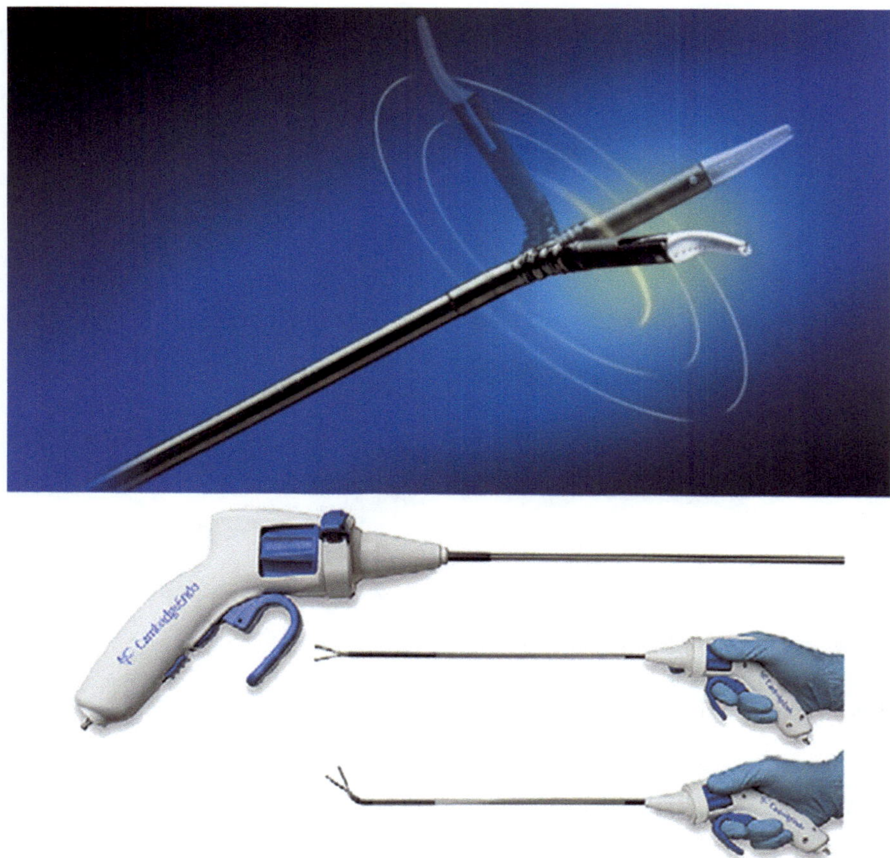

Fig. 6.14 Autonomy Laparo-Angle™ instruments

SILS™ Stitch instrument are designed to provide triangulation and visualization needed to facilitate laparoscopic surgery through a single incision.

6.1.3.4 SILS™ Hand Instruments (Covidien) (Fig. 6.16)

They provide a dynamic articulation allowing access to the surgical site from different angles by having handle moved off-axis. Main features include locking system, increased shaft length, 360° tip rotation, electrocautery connection.

6.1.3.5 Pre-bent Laparoscopic Instruments: S-PORTAL™ Series (Karl Storz) (Fig. 6.17) and HiQ LS™ Hand Instruments (Olympus) (Fig. 6.18)

These were developed to provide an optimal sheath curvature for some specific surgery, like cholecystectomy and appendectomy. Their relative simple design

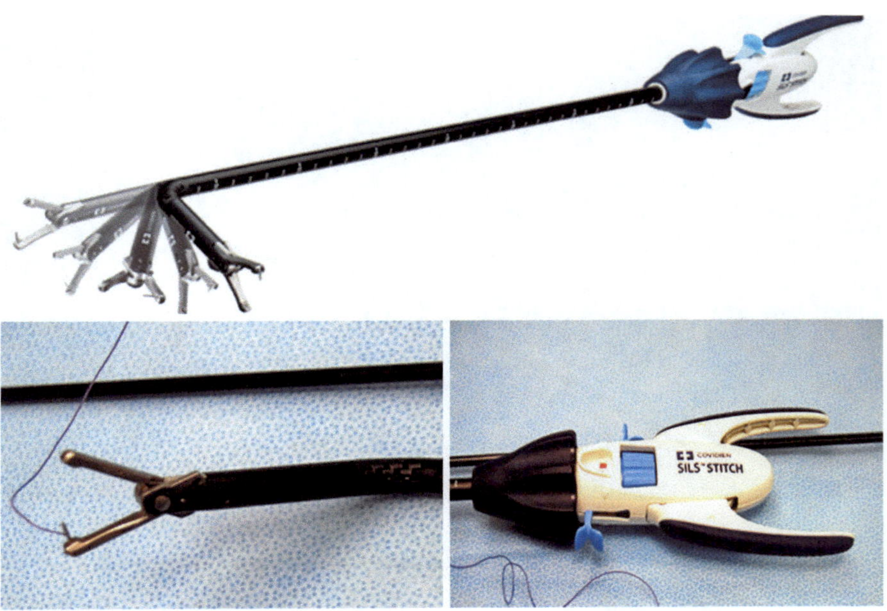

Fig. 6.15 SILS™ Stitch Articulating Endoscopic Suturing Device

Fig. 6.16 SILS™ Hand Instruments

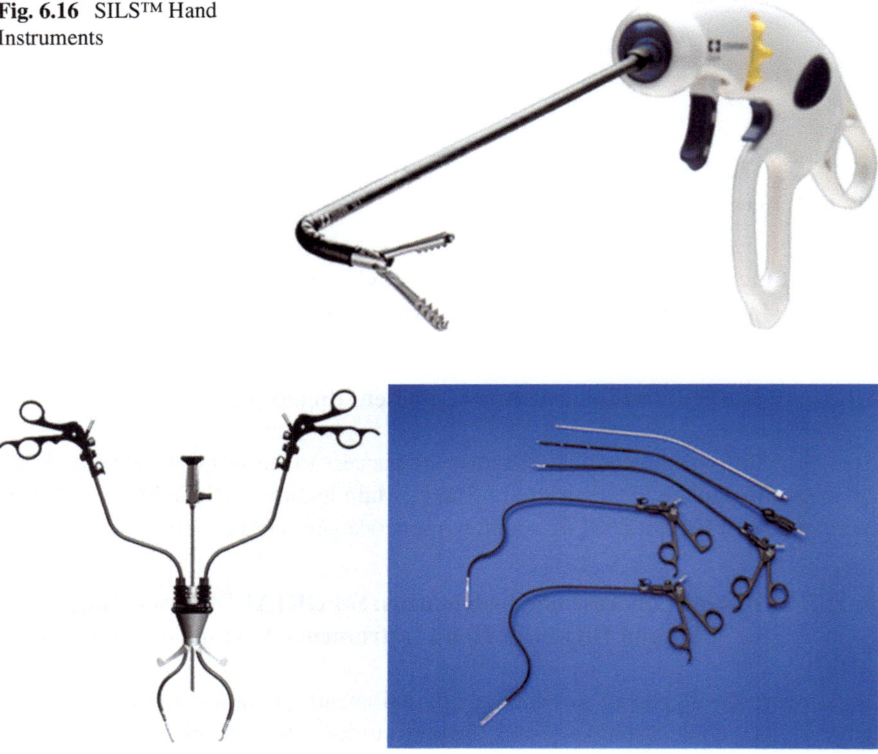

Fig. 6.17 Pre-bent laparoscopic instruments: S-PORTAL™ series

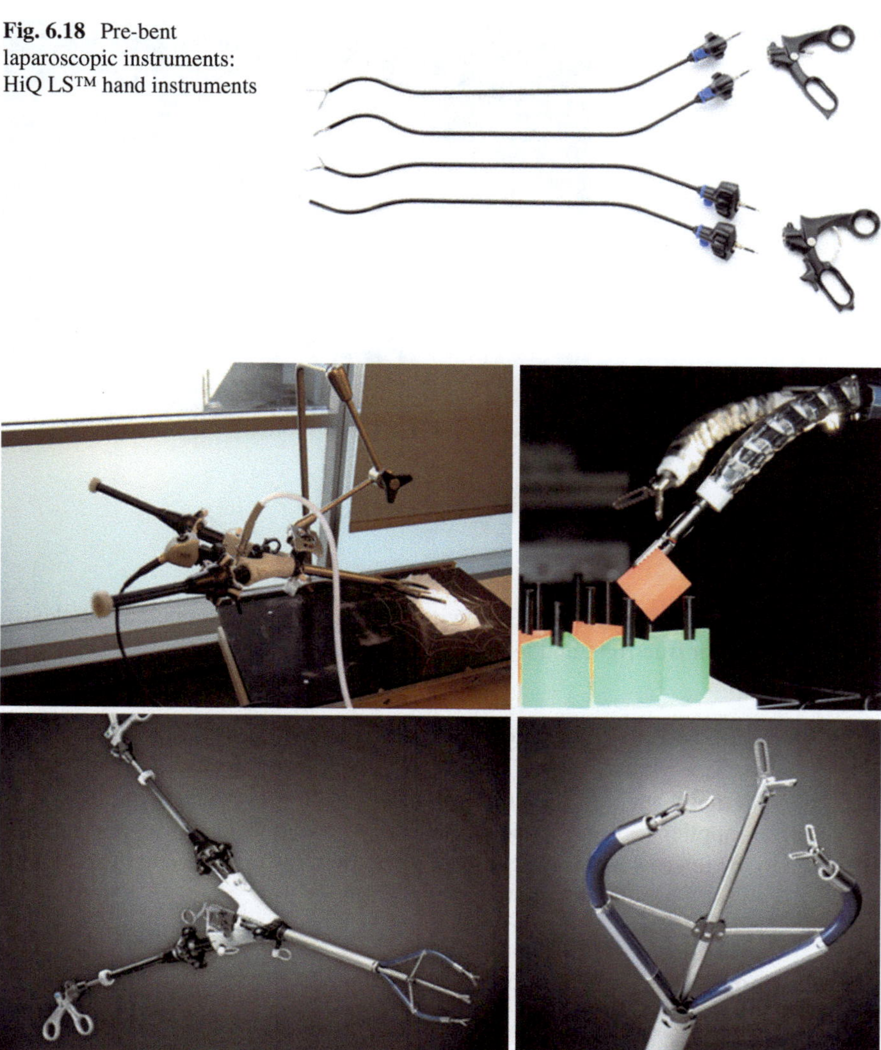

Fig. 6.18 Pre-bent laparoscopic instruments: HiQ LS™ hand instruments

Fig. 6.19 SPIDER™ Surgical System

ensures that the handles do not enter the operating range of the laparoscope and permits the surgeon to work in a comfortable, ergonomic position without the surgeon and camera assistant interfering with one another. However, for more complex urological surgery, their role, as compared to other disposable articulating instruments, remains to be determined.

6.1.3.6 SPIDER™ Surgical System (TransEnterix, Morrisville, USA) (Fig. 6.19)

This represents a novel platform specifically designed for LESS [14]. The unique design accommodates a range of flexible instruments through articulating instrument delivery tubes. Unlike early single port techniques, SPIDER eliminates the

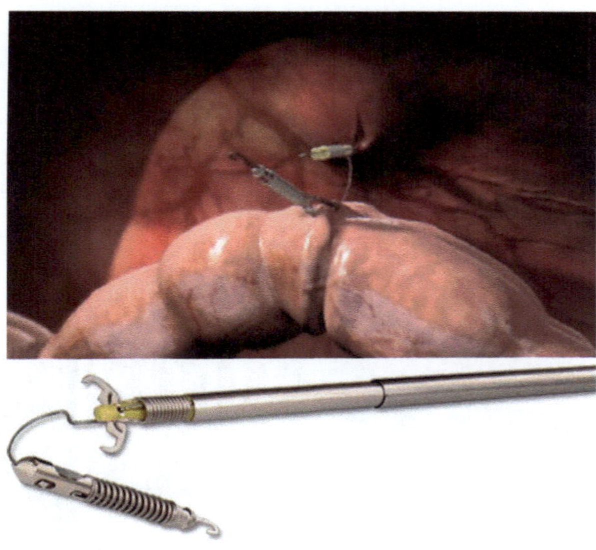

Fig. 6.20 EndoGrab™

awkward crossed arms movement, allowing a single surgeon to operate the device more naturally for true right and left instrument manipulation.

6.1.3.7 EndoGrab™ (Virtual Ports, Richmond, VA, USA) (Fig. 6.20)

This is an internally anchored, hands-free retracting device, which is introduced by means of an applier tool and attached to the organ requiring retraction, then be anchored to the internal abdominal wall. It can expose the operative field and eliminate the need for a handheld retractor during surgery.

6.1.3.8 EndoEYE™ LS (Olympus) (Fig. 6.21)

This is a 5-mm innovative laparoscope for the LESS. The all-in-one design integrates the light cable and camera system into the laparoscope for improved ergonomics and maintenance. It allows minimizing the clashing between the cable and the outside instruments.

6.1.3.9 EndoEYE LTF VP (Olympus) (Fig. 6.22)

This is a 5-mm novel all-in-one laparoscopy with the deflectable tip, which can provide a complete 100° field of view to visually capture the desired location head-on, from above, or from behind. This design allows the laparoscope to be placed to the side during the surgery, getting more space of the instruments.

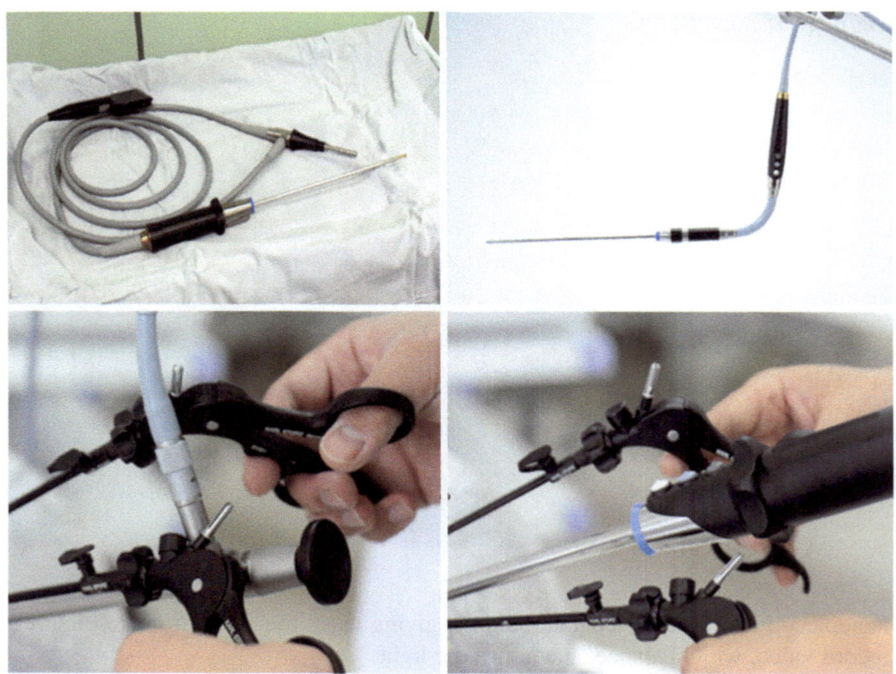

Fig. 6.21 To reduce the clashing using EndoEYE™ LS

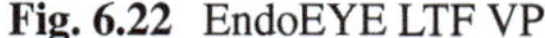

Fig. 6.22 EndoEYE LTF VP

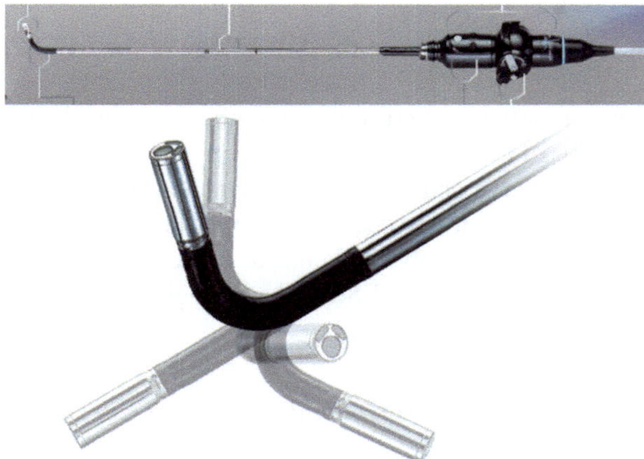

6.1.3.10 IDEAL EYES™ (Stryker) (Fig. 6.23)

This 10-mm novel articulating laparoscope with all-in one design includes distal flex tip technology to allow for 100° of flexion in all direction and transmits both HD (1,280 × 1,024) and HDTV (720p) video signals in the surgery. The ergonomic

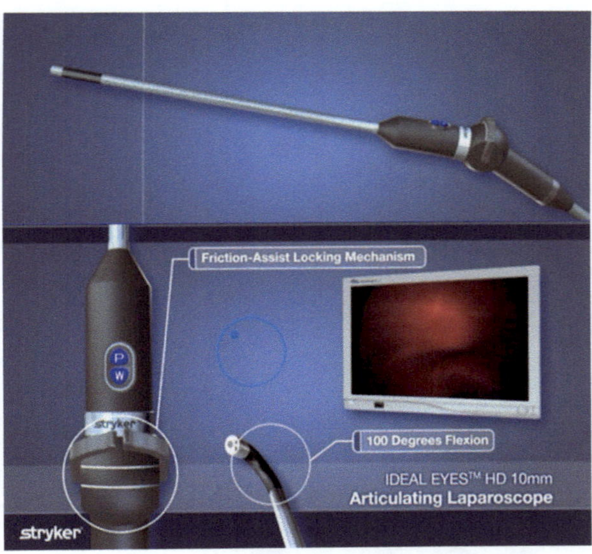

Fig. 6.23 IDEAL EYES™

handpiece includes two separate buttons, giving users the ability to take pictures, record video, white balance, and adjust the light.

6.1.4 The Challenges of the LESS

6.1.4.1 How to Prove the Advantage of the LESS?

Except for the cosmetic outcomes, objective data demonstrating the benefit of LESS in terms of less pain and faster recovery are not enough. When considering the steep learning curve and the poorly ergonomic operating setting, it becomes clear that stronger evidence is needed to ignite the passion of surgeons. Therefore, further prospective, possibly randomized, clinic studies are expected to define the actual place and benefits of LESS in the urologic armamentarium.

6.1.4.2 How to Overcome the Learning Curve of LESS?

As any novel and challenging technique, a critical issue is how to minimize the risk of complications during this initial stage. The successful previous experience with traditional laparoscopic surgery should serve as a reference, and different educational tools, including dry lab and hands-on animal labs and mentoring programs, should be adopted. By familiarizing with the novel flexible instruments and "cross-hand" operating mode, the surgeon should gain the necessary skills to perform a clinical case.

Besides this, the surgeon is expected to apply rigorous selection criteria to identify the most appropriate patient for LESS (e.g., low BMI, short shape, left kidney disease) in order to minimize the risk of the procedure. Operations without too many unexpected variables and not requiring a reconstructive part would represent the best choice for the novice LESS surgeon. Examples are renal cryotherapy, renal cyst decortication, and bilateral varicocele repair.

6.1.4.3 What Are the Tips and Tricks in LESS?

Triangulation represents a basic principle of laparoscopic surgery, and it can be restored during LESS by using articulating instruments. However, straight instruments are more effective for meticulous dissection. Thus, it is better to use one flexible instrument to retract or expose and one straight instrument to dissect the tissue (Fig. 6.24). A second tip to be adopted during LESS is the use of stay sutures or Hem-o-lok clips to anchor or suspend intra-abdominal structures (i.e., peritoneum, Gerota's fascia, renal pelvis, ureter) on the internal abdominal wall in order to achieve variable retraction and better exposure without adding extra ports (Fig. 6.25). The EndoGrab™ is another effective option for internal retraction.

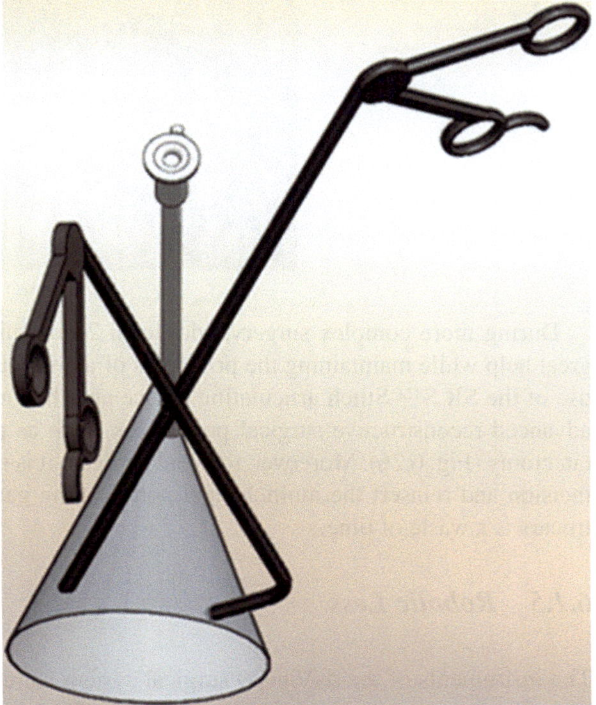

Fig. 6.24 The combination of the straight and articulating instruments in LESS

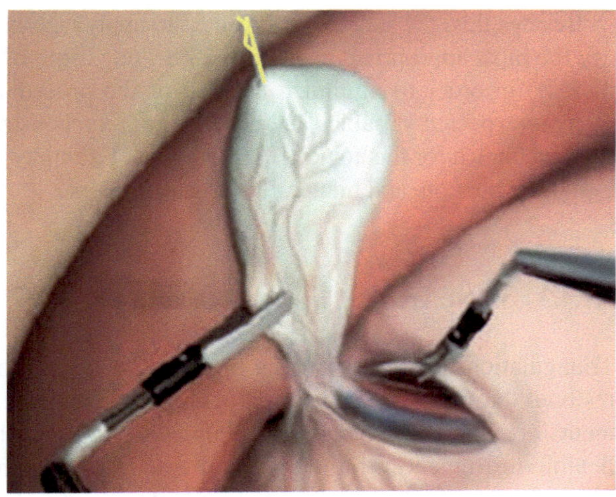

Fig. 6.25 To place the stay sutures in LESS

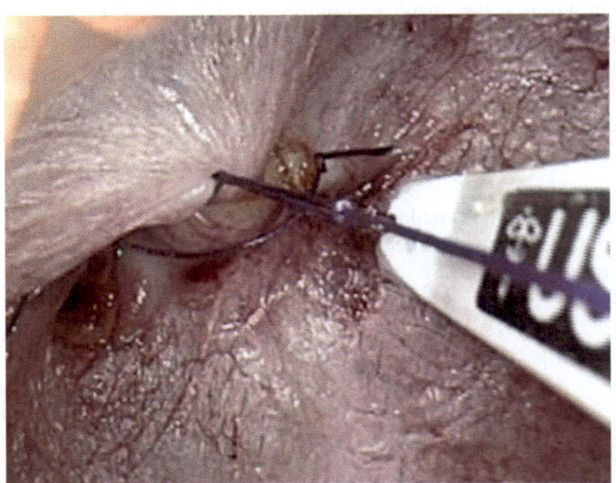

Fig. 6.26 To push the knot in the complex surgery

During more complex surgery, additional 2-mm mini-instruments can provide great help while maintaining the principles of a minimal trauma. Another tip is the use of the SILS™ Stitch articulating device and the knot pusher when performing advanced reconstructive surgical procedures, such as pyeloplasty or radical prostatectomy (Fig. 6.26). Moreover, to avoid gas leak, it is important to close part of the incision and reinsert the multichannel port. Putting gauze or materials around the trocars is a waste of time.

6.1.5 Robotic Less

The instruments of the daVinci® surgical system (Intuitive Surgical) are designed with 7° of motion that mimic the dexterity of the human hand and wrist. This inherent feature of the robotic arm provides superior ergonomics when performing LESS, especially for complex reconstructive surgery.

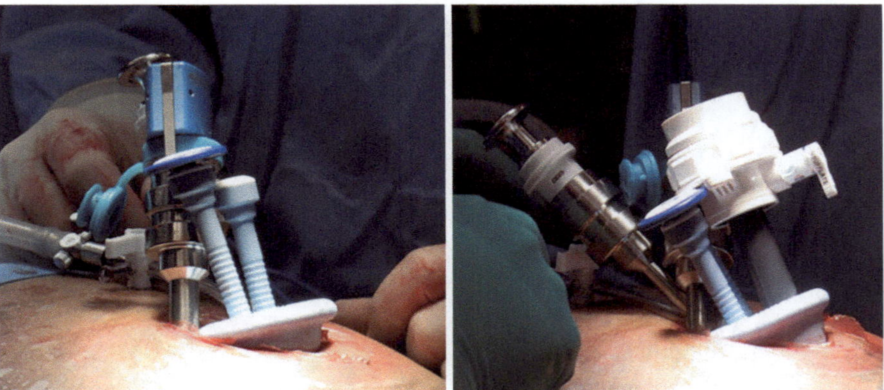

Fig. 6.27 The line configuration of SILS and robotic ports in robotic LESS

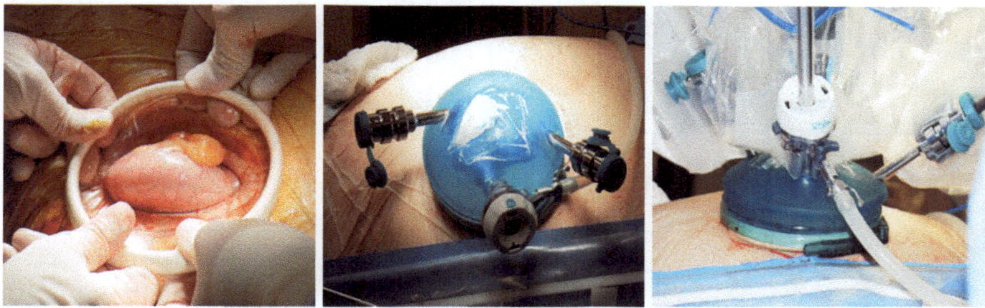

Fig. 6.28 The GelPort in robotic LESS

After an initial experience in the animal lab, robotic LESS has been proved to be feasible for a variety of urological surgeries. Kaouk et al. [15] first reported the initial clinical experience with robotic LESS in 2009, describing pyeloplasty, radical nephrectomy, and radical prostatectomy.

The abdominal access for robotic LESS procedures is gained by placing additional one or two 8-mm robotic ports alongside the multichannel port in the same skin incision (Fig. 6.27). This novel configuration of port is effective in reducing the instrument clashing and mechanical restrictions without additional incision.

For procedures where the removal of a larger specimen is expected, such as radical nephrectomy or donor nephrectomy, the GelPort™ can provide more space and flexibility for the robotic port placement due to a larger skin incision (Fig. 6.28).

However, when dissecting at the upper or low pole of the operating field, the movement of the bulky robotic arm is obviously limited because of the frequent clashing.

Recently, an innovation for the daVinci® surgical system has been developed to overcome the current technical challenges of robotic LESS, the so-called VeSPA instruments [16].

Using a crossing configuration and a special multichannel port, the robotic arm can avoid any crowding (Fig. 6.29). With the help of modern computer technology, the surgeon can control the instrument in the same way of the standard daVinci LESS but with the advantage of improved ergonomics (Fig. 6.30).

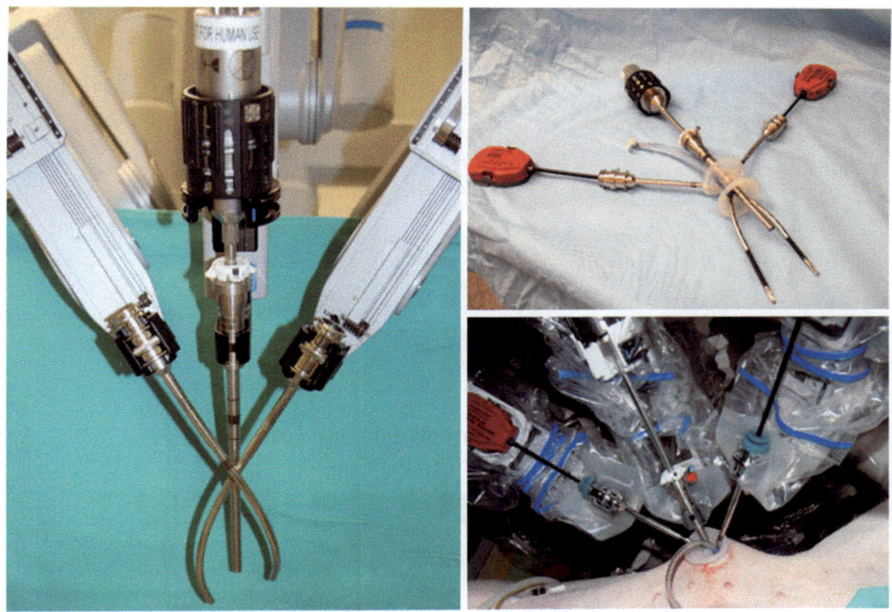

Fig. 6.29 The novel single port robotic surgical system (VeSPA)

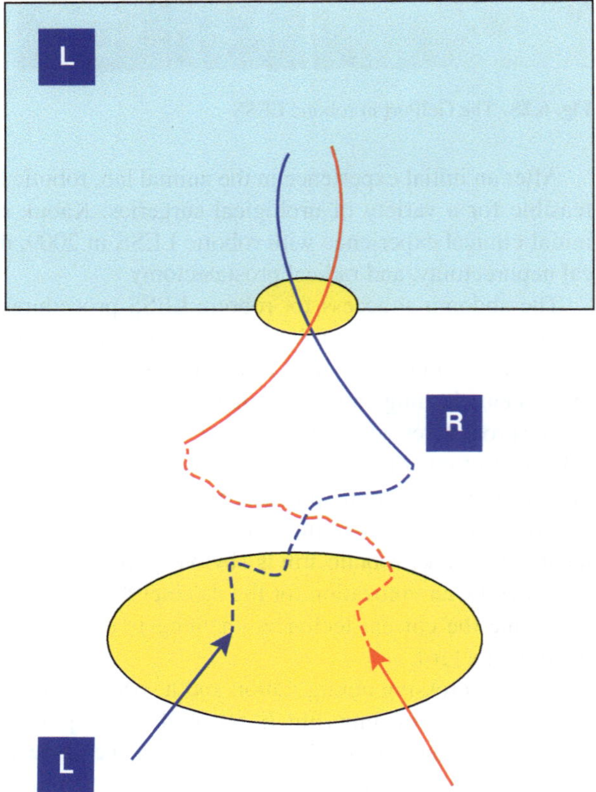

Fig. 6.30 The signal transduction pathway of the VeSPA

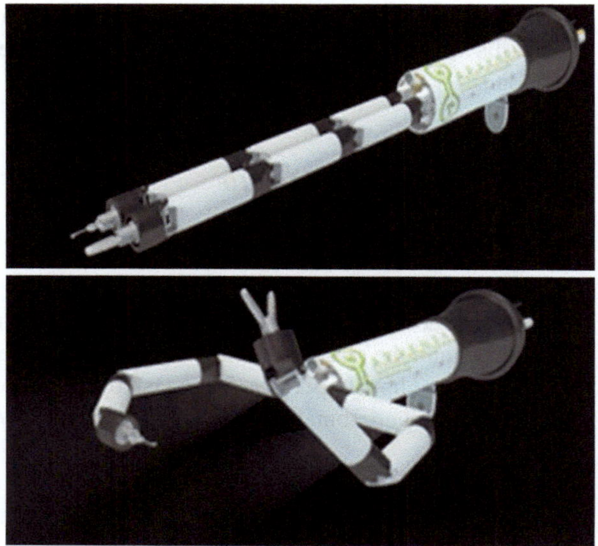

Fig. 6.31 The future mini-robotic platform: ARAKNES

Haber et al. [16] reported the first experience of the animal lab, including simple nephrectomy, partial nephrectomy, and pyeloplasty. All 16 procedures were performed successfully without the addition of ports or open conversion. With VeSPA, the robotic arm does not provide the full range of motion given by the EndoWrist™ technology, which can be a disadvantage when performing reconstructive surgery.

Some imaginative innovations in the field of robotic LESS are still in the early experimental stage. An interesting example is the ARAKNES project. This is a mini-robotic platform that can be introduced into abdomen and, once there, unfolded to operate (Fig. 6.31).

This and other ongoing projects are expected to overcome the current limitations for LESS.

6.2 Training Module for Basic Skill in LESS

6.2.1 Introduction

With the increasing use of the LESS in urology, appropriate training programs need to be established to allow urologic surgeons to master this new technology.

Notably, LESS is technically more challenging than standard laparoscopy. However, specialized training courses for LESS are rarely available. Basic traditional laparoscopic training exercises may not be suitable for training in LESS as this new technique has features, such as poor triangulation, difficult retraction, instrument crowding, and in-line vision.

To address this issue, we designed a specialized course for training in LESS basic skills with technical challenges similar to those encountered during a LESS operation.

6.2.2 *The Training Module*

6.2.2.1 Learning Objectives

- To become accustomed to flexible/articulating instruments
- To understand the clashing phenomenon between the instruments and the scope
- To understand how to perform basic task by using the crossing method
- To try different combinations of straight and flexible/articulating instruments

6.2.2.2 Station Setup

- Semicircular-shaped simulator
- 5-mm EndoEYE™ LS or EndoEYE LTF VP (Olympus)
- Multichannel port (TriPort™, Olympus)
- Standard laparoscopic instruments, including Maryland forceps and scissors
- Flexible laparoscopic instruments (Autonomy Laparo-Angle™ series), including Maryland forceps and scissors.

6.2.2.3 Description of the Training Procedure

- Step 1: Z-shaped line cut (Fig. 6.32)
- The plastic fixators are deployed in a "Z" shape on a multiporous plastic plaque, and connecting rubber bands are placed between fixators. The trainee is required to cut the bands off with the common grasper and the 5-mm flexible scissors in turn in a "Z" shape.

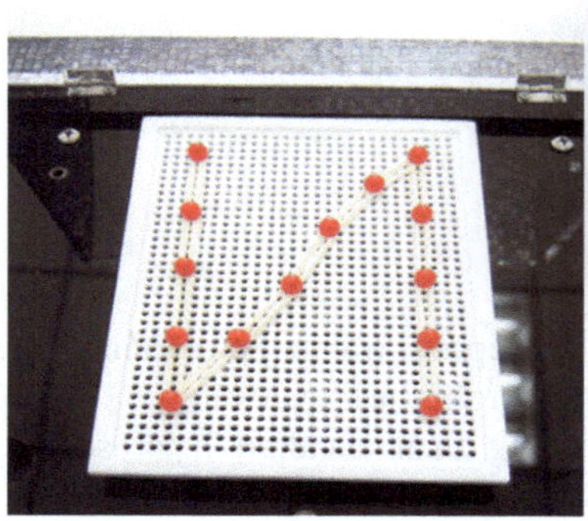
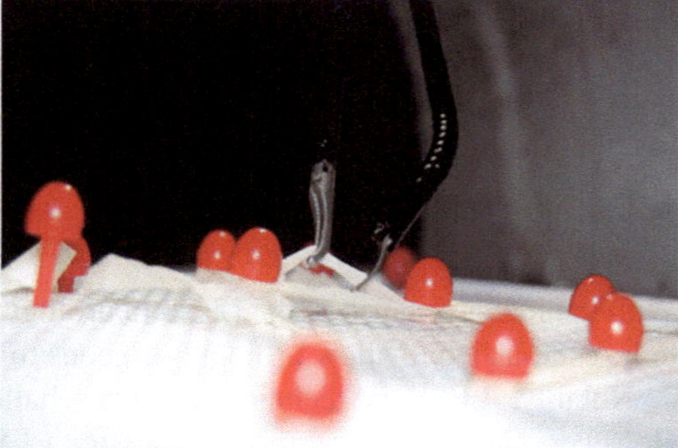

Fig. 6.32 To cut the line in a "Z" shape

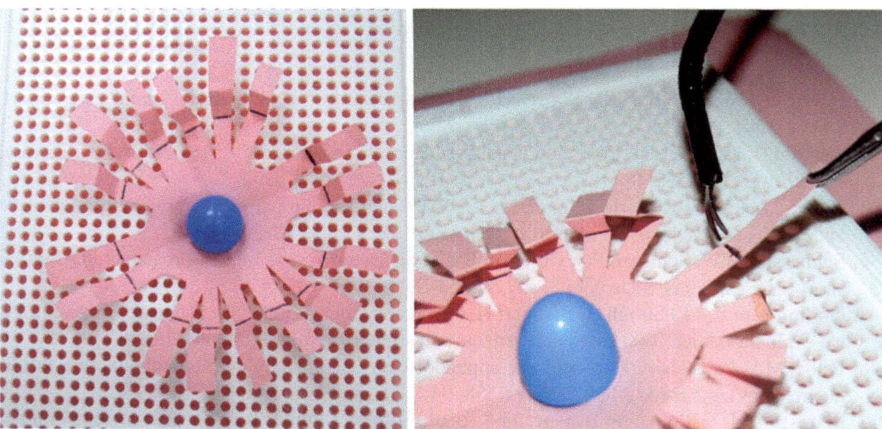

Fig. 6.33 To cut "petaloid"-folded slips

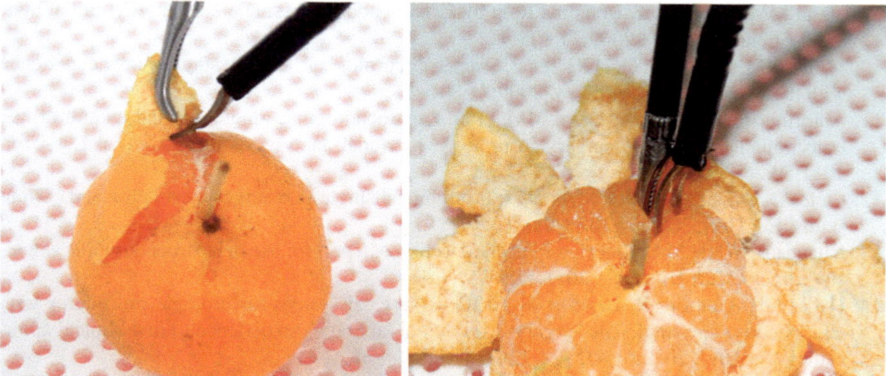

Fig. 6.34 To dissect the orange

- Step 2: Petal-shaped paper cut (Fig. 6.33)
- A piece of round paper with the radius of 5 cm is cut into a "petaloid" shape and then threefolded with lines on the inner one-third folded section. The paper is then fixed on the center of a multiporous plastic plaque with plastic fixators. The trainee is required to stretch petals with the common grasper in the left hand and then cut the "petaloid" folded slips along the lines with the flexible scissors in the right hand.
- Step 3: Peeling orange (Fig. 6.34)
- An orange is fixed on the center of a multiporous plastic plaque with a toothpick. Then, as previously described in Chap. 3, the orange should be peeled and its segments separated with the common grasper and the flexible scissor. During the exercise, the trainee can adopt different combination of straight or flexible instruments.

References

1. Clayman RV, Kavoussi LR, Soper NJ, et al. Laparoscopic nephrectomy: initial case report. J Urol. 1991;146:278.
2. Jonsson B, Zethraeus N. Costs and benefits of laparoscopic surgery – a review of the literature. Eur J Surg. 2000;585:48.
3. Kaul S, Laungani R, Sarle R, et al. da Vinci-assisted robotic partial nephrectomy: technique and results at a mean of 15 months of follow-up. Eur Urol. 2007;51:186–91.
4. Schuessler WW, Schulam PG, Clayman RV, et al. Laparoscopic radical prostatectomy: initial short-term experience. Urology. 1997;50:854–7.
5. Guillonneau B, El-Fettouh H, Baumert H, et al. Laparoscopic radical prostatectomy: oncological evaluation after 1000 cases at Montsouris Institute. J Urol. 2003;169:1261–6.
6. Pelosi MA, Pelosi MA. Laparoscopic appendectomy using a single umbilical puncture (minilaparoscopy). J Reprod Med. 1992;37:588–94.
7. Marescaux J, Dallemagne B, Perretta S, et al. Surgery without scars: report of transluminal cholecystectomy in a human being. Arch Surg. 1997;142:823–6.
8. Rane A, Rao PP, Rao SP, et al. Clinical evaluation of a novel laparoscopic port (R-Port TM) in urology and evolution of the single laparoscopic port procedure (SLAPP). J Endourol. 2007; Abstract BR6-01.
9. Desai MM, Berger AK, Brandina R, et al. Laparoendoscopic single-site surgery: initial hundred patients. Urology. 2009;74:805–12.
10. White WM, Haber GP, Goel RK, et al. Single-port urological surgery: single-center experience with the first 100 cases. Urology. 2009;74:801–4.
11. Autorino R, Cadeddu JA, Desai MM, et al. Laparoendoscopic single-site and natural orifice transluminal endoscopic surgery in urology: a critical analysis of the literature. Eur Urol. 2011;59:26–45.
12. Canes D, Desai MM, Aron M, et al. Transumbilical single-port surgery: evolution and current status. Eur Urol. 2008;54:1020–9.
13. Khanna R, White MA, Autorino R, et al. Selection of a port for use in laparoendoscopic single-site surgery. Curr Urol Rep. 2011;12:94–9.
14. Haber GP, Autorino R, Laydner H. SPIDER surgical system for urologic procedures with laparoendoscopic single-site surgery: from initial laboratory experience to first clinical application. Eur Urol. 2012;61:415–22. Epub ahead of print.
15. White MA, Autorino R, Spana G, et al. Robotic laparoendoscopic single-site radical nephrectomy: surgical technique and comparative outcomes. Eur Urol. 2011;59:815–22.
16. Haber GP, White MA, Autorino R, et al. Novel robotic da Vinci instruments for laparoendoscopic single-site surgery. Urology. 2010;76:1279–82.

Chapter 7
Skills and Training Course in Robotic Laparoscopic Urology

Ananthakrishnan Sivaraman, Rafael F. Coelho, Sanket Chauhan, Kenneth J. Palmer, and Vipul R. Patel

Abstract Yesterday's humor is today's reality. Robotic surgery provides the minimal invasiveness of laparoscopy with better precision, more freedom of motion, and lack of tremor. The initial step of training protocol for proficiency and credentialing in robot-assisted surgery would be skills on operating the robot in labs and then progressing onto mastery of procedure-specific nuances. Proctoring and preceptoring are two different but indispensible approaches to converting the laboratory and simulation expertise into operative ability. The training of the support team including the theater staff and first assistant is another important aspect of achieving proficiency and optimal outcomes in robotic urology. Ethical issues and cost factors limit the widespread use of robots in the training program.

Keywords Robotic surgery • Urology • Laparoscopy • Training course • Radical prostatectomy

---

A. Sivaraman, M.S., MCh, DNB, FRCS (Urol) • S. Chauhan, M.D. • K.J. Palmer, M.D.
V.R. Patel, M.D. (✉)
Department of Urology, Global Robotics Institute, Florida Hospital Celebration Health,
410 Celebration Place, STE 200, Celebration, FL 34747, USA
e-mail: vipul.patel.md@flhosp.org

R.F. Coelho, M.D.
Department of Urology, Global Robotics Institute, Florida Hospital Celebration Health,
410 Celebration Place, STE 200, Celebration, FL 34747, USA

Departmento do Urologia,
Hospital Israelita Albert Einstein, São Paulo, Brazil

Instituto do Câncer do Estado de São Paulo,
São Paulo, Brazil

Cardeal Arcoverde 201 apt 143, São Paulo 05407000, Brazil

Y.H. Sun et al. (eds.), *The Training Courses of Urological Laparoscopy*,
DOI 10.1007/978-1-4471-2723-9_7, © Springer-Verlag London 2012

7.1 Introduction

Robotic surgery has established itself as a major advance in the last 10 years. The advantages of this technique have been well documented in urological practice with the majority of radical prostatectomy in the United States being done with robotic assistance [1].

The introduction of any innovative technology in surgery is associated with a time period when surgeons develop the knowledge and skills required to perform the procedure safely and efficiently. This time period is generally referred to as the learning curve. One of the claimed benefits of the robot-assisted approach is a shortening of the protracted learning curve associated with laparoscopic radical prostatectomy that has prevented the widespread adoption of this minimally invasive approach by most urologic surgeons. Initial reports on the learning curve for robotic-assisted laparoscopic radical prostatectomy (RARP) suggested that <20 cases are required for the surgeon to acquire basic proficiency with the procedure [2]. However, with increasing experience and standardization of the surgical technique, it has become evident that far greater experience is required for the surgeon to be confident and proficient, providing patients with high-quality perioperative, functional, and oncologic outcomes as demonstrated by Vickers et al. [3].

The resources required for robotic surgery are however high [4], and it becomes essential that the utilization of the daVinci system is maximized to make the technique economically viable. Although robotic programs the world over are currently centered on radical prostatectomy, the indications for this technique will be gradually expanded to make the heavy investment economically justifiable. It will also be required that the results of RARP as measured by the trifecta outcomes be significantly better than conventional laparoscopy and open surgery on a consistent basis. This will require structured training and mentoring for the surgeon aiming to master this technique.

This chapter will discuss the two key issues of training protocol for proficiency, credentialing in robot-assisted surgery and the surgical steps in robotic-assisted radical prostatectomy with modifications needed to achieve good outcomes.

7.2 Training in Robotic Urology

Proper guidelines on training and credentialing of surgeons and institutions do not exist. Any training protocol should address patient safety and physician liability as key issues. We present here our views on training in urological robotic surgery.

The robot is to be considered a means to an end, and the end result is achieving optimal surgical outcomes for the patient. The robot does have its limitations, and in recognizing it the surgeon can use it to his advantage. "The aircraft is only as good as the pilot," and hence, the surgeon's foundation on basic principles of surgery should be strong before embarking on robotic training. Currently, the robot is still considered as an advanced surgical tool and as such does not figure in basic surgical training. However, this situation may change in future with robotic training being included in the curriculum for residents as well as a number of short-term courses being conducted on robotic training.

The transition from open and laparoscopic surgery to robot-assisted surgery does have a learning curve [2]. For the robotically naïve urologist or trainee, developing sufficient robotic skills requires extensive training. It involves a structured training program to acquire robotic skills and proficiency in minimally invasive procedures based on the basic surgical principles used in open and laparoscopic surgery but on a robotic interface. It should not only encompass mastering the surgical robotic technology but create an understanding of the instrument, the electronic and mechanical components, be able to acquire baseline knowledge to troubleshoot all parts of the system, master surgical telemanipulation as applied to specific surgical procedures, and hone skills as a facile patient side assistant. Training should be considered as a journey that includes a blend of computer-based training, simulation, laboratory experience, and hands-on experience with the help of proctoring.

"Repetition is the mother of skill." Surgical practice makes perfect, but with the help of better training tools, the learning curve can be shortened without compromising the welfare of the patient. The initial step would be skills on operating the robot and then progressing onto mastery of procedure-specific nuances. Dry and wet lab training is the first step toward acquiring the requisite skill set. Achieving proficiency in hand-eye coordination, the utilization of the clutch, movement of the camera, etc., would require performing repetitive exercises in the dry lab. Skill-specific models are commercially available for various exercises [5]. Cadaver and animal labs have a unique place in training because of their ability to produce an environment that mimics live surgery accurately. However, ethical issues and cost factors limit their widespread use. Medicolegal pressures and mandates for cost-effective performance have popularized surgical simulation training that provides a more realistic experience with an element of haptic feedback. Simulators as tools of procedural training and credentialing allow hours of practice and help the surgeon learn from mistakes. These simulators come with inbuilt software that calculates the accuracy of the surgeon, time taken, and economy of motion and gives out a comprehensive report. There are currently several high quality simulators in the market [6, 7]. With more teaching institutions investing in simulators and mini-resident courses offered on robotic training, it can only result in increased benefits to the patient. Additionally, there are several dedicated robotic training labs currently offering basic and advanced course on robotic surgery [8].

When technology meets expertise, great results can be achieved. So also in the case of Robotic surgery, the robot is only a technological tool in the hands of the surgeon. Hence, it is very important that the surgeon undergoes procedure-specific training, as each surgery will have specific nuances that have to be mastered. To be able to handle complications is another important chip toward patient well-being. This can be achieved by shadowing an experienced surgeon in centers of excellence or by doing fellowships in robotic surgery. The port placement, operating room setup, and the relative roles of the assistant can also be learned in this stint. Converting the laboratory and simulation expertise into operative ability is not always easy and requires the assistance of a mentor. This part of the learning curve is overcome by access to an expert surgeon for proctoring and preceptoring.

Until recently, residencies did not have robotics, and even so, the experience the surgeons gain greatly varies depending upon the program and specialty. Robotic fellowship programs have been started in recent years, but again, it is specialty specific. An initial period of supervision is mandatory for proper development of knowledge and skills in a trainee surgeon. In order to produce consistent results, a standardization of procedure needs to be developed. So also in the case of robotic training, a standardized credentialing system needs to be in place to evaluate surgeon competency and safety with robotic urological performance. Proctoring is a modality that can be used to achieve this.

Proctoring and preceptoring are two different approaches to training [1]. Proctoring involves an expert surgeon observing and assessing the skills and knowledge of the surgeon in training with a view to making recommendations regarding further training or privileging. The proctor is not liable for the well-being of the patient being operated upon. A preceptor takes a more hands-on approach and supervises the surgeon in training and if need arises, takes over the surgery. The ultimate responsibility of the patient's well-being rests with the preceptor. The time duration of preceptoring and proctoring is not clearly defined but should vary according to the individual's ability to master a given procedure.

The preceptor and trainee may work together, or the learning experience may be part of a fellowship or residency. Preceptors or experienced robotic surgeons can also travel to the institution initiating the robotic program. This involves practical difficulties for the preceptor with regard to time and travel. Advanced technology has opened new avenues for long-distance observation through teleproctoring. Although still in its infancy, telesurgery can be used to train surgeons in robotic techniques and be used for consultations and telementoring. Telemedicine can overcome some of the practical difficulties. With the help of this technology, an expert surgeon stationed remotely can supervise a trainee from his place of work.

A recent landmark initiative by McDougall et al. [9] was the establishment of a comprehensive 5-day mini-residency program at the University of California at Irvine in 2003. The residency program included dry lab, animal and cadaver laboratory skills training, and live demonstrations in the operating room. All participants in the course were robotically naive but laparoscopically experienced. Within 14 months of the program, 95% were successfully performing RARP. Several reports have shown the presence of a significant learning curve ranging from 20 to 100 cases for RARP [2, 10, 11]. With a structured training program, this number will eventually be brought down to acceptable levels. No patient wants to be part of a surgeon learning curve, and it is incumbent on the trainers to reduce the learning curve of trainees as much as possible.

Another important aspect of achieving proficiency and optimal outcomes is the training of the support team including the theater staff and first assistant [12]. Contrary to traditional open surgery, robotic surgery implies that the leading surgeon does not have direct contact with the patient being completely immersed in the console, and the scrub nurse (SN) and physician assistant (PA) are the only ones in direct contact with the patient. A complete understanding of the procedure and the surgical steps is crucial. The scrub nurse should coordinate with the PA during the entire procedure, providing sutures and instruments and helping taking care of the camera.

A scarce coordination between PA and SN can cause significant delays and difficulties during the procedure. As robotic surgery currently is a team effort, results are directly reflective of all members of the team. The key members of the core surgical team need to be trained in all the steps of the surgery being performed. Each of the members of the team should know what exactly is required of them and at what time frames of the procedure.

7.3 Robot-Assisted Radical Prostatectomy

Data from the Surveillance, Epidemiology and End Results (SEER) registry indicate that prostate cancer forms 28% of newly diagnosed cancers in men [13]. For patients with organ-confined disease, numerous treatment alternatives are now available. However, since Walsh et al. first introduced the anatomic nerve-sparing technique for radical prostatectomy (RP), it has become the gold standard and most widespread treatment for clinically localized prostate cancer, providing excellent long cancer control. More recently, with the introduction of robotic technology in the field of urology and the pioneering work of Binder and Krammer [14], robot-assisted radical prostatectomy has made rapid advances in the last decade.

Once the team acquires a level of proficiency and the robotic program is underway, the next significant improvement in outcomes will be due to incorporation of procedure-specific nuances and refinements. In this section, we explain our technique of robotic-assisted radical prostatectomy. This technique has evolved over a period of years and incorporates several modifications, which are essential to achieve optimal outcomes.

RALP can be performed via a transperitoneal or preperitoneal technique (Table 7.1). The transperitoneal approach is the most commonly utilized and is also the preferred method of the authors. The peritoneal cavity can be accessed by using either a Veress needle or Hasson technique, and the abdomen is then insufflated to a maximum pressure of 15 mmHg. Six trocars are placed under direct vision, as shown in Fig.7.1. The patient is then placed in a 25-degree steep Trendelenburg position and the robot docked.

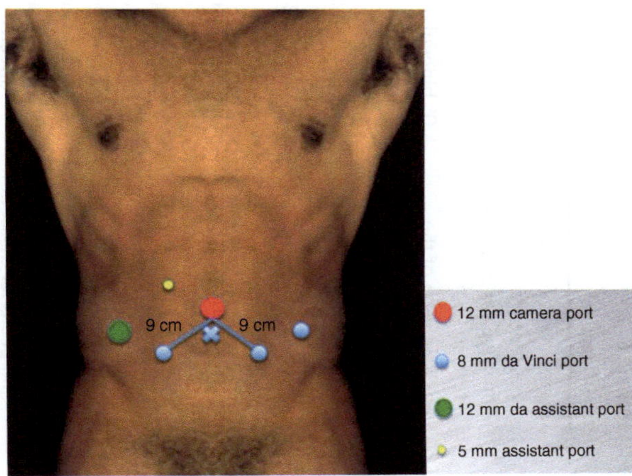

Fig. 7.1 Port placement

Table 7.1 RALP surgical steps

Surgical step	Lens	Right robotic instrument	Left robotic instrument	Fourth robotic arm	Assistant port
Step 1: Incision of the peritoneum and entry into the retropubic space of retzius	0° binocular lens	Monopolar scissor (25 W)	PK (plasma kinetic) forceps (26 W)	Prograsp	Microfrance grasper and suction
Step 2: Incision of the endopelvic fascia (EPF) and identification of the dorsal venous complex (DVC)	0° binocular lens	Monopolar scissor (25 W)	PK (plasma kinetic) forceps (26 W)	Prograsp	Grasper and suction
Step 3: Ligation of the DVC and Periurethral	0° binocular lens	Robotic needle driver	Robotic needle driver	Prograsp	Laparoscopic scissor and suction
Step 4: Anterior bladder neck dissection	30° binocular lens directed downward	Monopolar scissor (25 W)	PK (plasma kinetic) forceps (26 W)	Prograsp	Microfrance grasper and suction
Step 5: Posterior bladder neck dissection	30° binocular lens directed downwards	Monopolar scissor (25 W)	PK (plasma kinetic) forceps (26 W)	Prograsp	Microfrance grasper and suction
Step 6: Athermal Seminal vesicle dissection	30° binocular lens directed downwards	Monopolar scissor (25 W)	PK (plasma kinetic) forceps (26 W)	Prograsp	Microfrance grasper and suction
Step 7: Denonvillier's fascia and posterior dissection	30° binocular lens directed downwards	Monopolar scissor (25 W	PK (plasma kinetic) forceps (26 W)	Prograsp	Microfrance grasper and suction
Step 8: Nerve-sparing: "Athermal early retrograde release of the neurovascular bundle"	30° binocular lens directed downwards	Monopolar scissor (25 W)	PK (plasma kinetic) forceps (26 W)	Prograsp	Microfrance grasper and suction
Step 9: Apical dissection	30° binocular lens directed downwards	Monopolar scissor (25 W)	PK (plasma kinetic) forceps (26 W)	Prograsp	Microfrance grasper and suction
Step 10: Modified posterior reconstruction of the rhabdosphincter and urethrovesical anastomosis	30° binocular lens directed downwards	Robotic needle driver	Robotic needle driver	Prograsp	Suction and scissor

7.3.1 *Peritoneal Incision and Entry into the Space of Retzius*

An inverted U-shaped incision is made through the median umbilical ligament and is extended to the vas deferens on both sides. The peritoneum is dissected from the pubic bone superiorly, the median umbilical ligaments laterally, and the vas deferens inferolaterally. Peritoneal dissection needs to be carried all the way to the base of the vas in order to effectively free the bladder. Key steps are identification of the pubic tubercle and carrying the dissection laterally to the vas. Traction and countertraction are essential and provided by the assistant and the fourth arm.

7.3.2 *Incision of the Endopelvic Fascia (EPF)*

The incision of the EPF is best done at the base of the prostate. The levator muscles are gently separated from the prostate with the aid of the scissors used to incise the endopelvic fascia. The incision on the EPF is carried toward the apex of the prostate separating the levator muscles from the prostate until the apex of the prostate is reached. After adequate exposure, the endopelvic fascia is opened immediately, lateral to the puboprostatic ligaments bilaterally. As the levator fibers are pushed away, the dorsal venous complex and the urethra come into view (Fig. 7.2).

7.3.3 *Ligation of the DVC and Periurethral Suspension Stitch*

The DVC is ligated using a 0 Caprosyn suture on a CT1 needle. The needle is held 2/3 from the tip at a downward angle and is placed in the visible notch between the urethra and the DVC. It is initially pushed across at 90° and then curved around the apex of the prostate using a slip knot. A slip knot is preferable because it prevents loosening of the suture as it is tied.

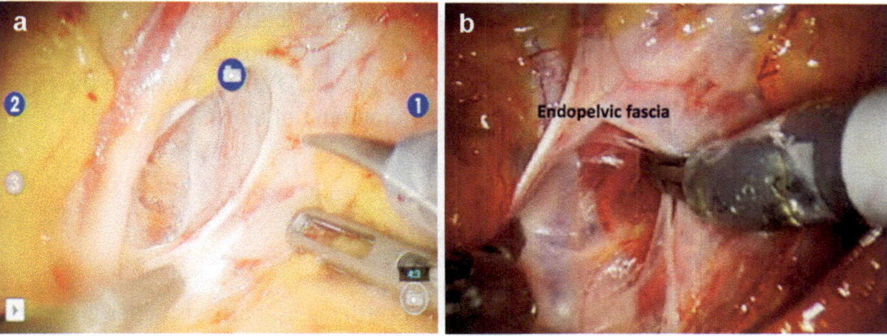

Fig. 7.2 Incision of the endopelvic fascia. (**a**) Exposure of endopelvic fascia (**b**) To push away levator fibers from the prostate surface

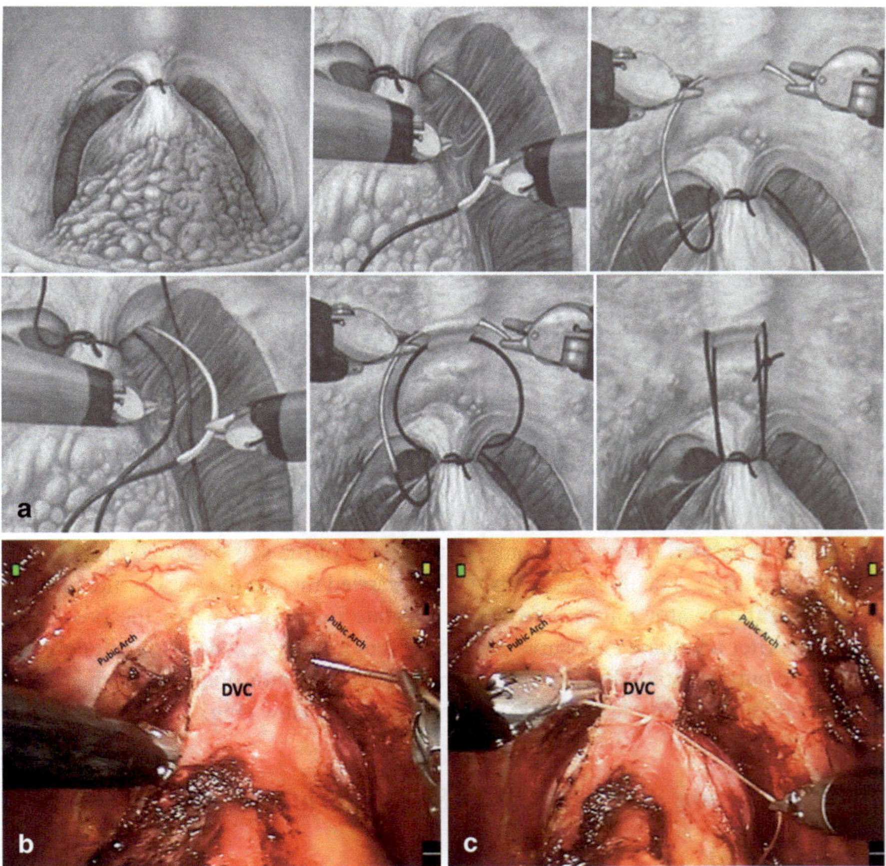

Fig. 7.3 Ligation of the DVC and periurethral suspension stitch. (**a**) To place a periurethral retropubic suspension. (**b**) To pass the CT1 needle between the plane of urethra and DVC. (**c**) Ligation of the DVC

A periurethral retropubic suspension stitch is then placed. This stitch is positioned holding the needle two-thirds of the way back in a 90°angle and passed from right side to left between the urethra and DVC, and then through the periosteum on the pubic bone. The stitch is passed again through the DVC and through the pubic bone, in a figure eight, and then tied with mild amount of tension (Fig. 7.3).

7.3.4 Anterior Bladder Neck Dissection

For this part of the surgery, a 30-degree lens is utilized as it affords better visualization of the bladder neck. The prostatovesical junction is identified as the area of cessation of the fat extending from the bladder (Fig. 7.4). Another method to identify the junction would be to pull on the urethral Foley catheter and see the balloon

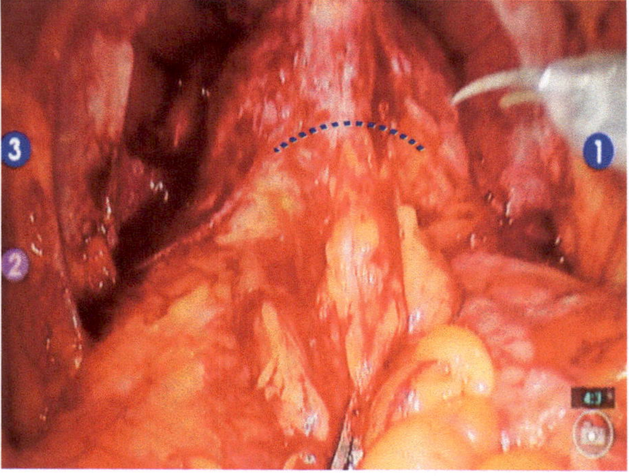

Fig. 7.4 Anterior bladder neck dissection – the urinary catheter is pulled and the prostatovesical junction is identified

hitch against the prostate. This technique may be misleading in the presence of large median lobes or previous TURP. The anterior bladder neck is incised with monopolar scissors cautery. The incision is started in the midline using a sweeping motion of the monopolar scissors while visualizing the bladder fibers. The key is to stick to the midline till the bladder neck is opened and then dissect laterally so as to avoid the lateral venous sinuses. Once the anterior urethra is divided, the fourth arm is used to grasp the Foley catheter and provide upward traction and expose the posterior bladder neck.

7.3.5 Posterior Bladder Neck Dissection

The posterior bladder neck is incised at the junction between the prostate and the bladder (Fig. 7.5). The lip of the posterior bladder neck is grasped with the Maryland dissector, and further dissection is carried out in a cephalad direction. The key points here are the appreciation and maintenance of the posterior tissue plane between the bladder and the prostate and proceeding with dissection in a cephalad direction so as to identify the seminal vesicles. The depth and direction of this dissection are important because there is a possibility of missing the seminal vesicles. The lateral bladder attachments to the prostate are controlled with Hem-o-lok clips.

7.3.6 Seminal Vesical Dissection

Accurate identification of the plane between the bladder and the prostate and further dissection in a cephalad manner expose the seminal vesicle and the vas. The thin fascial layers over the seminal vesicles and vas are open. The fourth arm is used to retract the vas superiorly, and it is incised. The inferior portion of the vas is retracted by the assistant, and the vas is followed posteriorly to expose the tip of the seminal

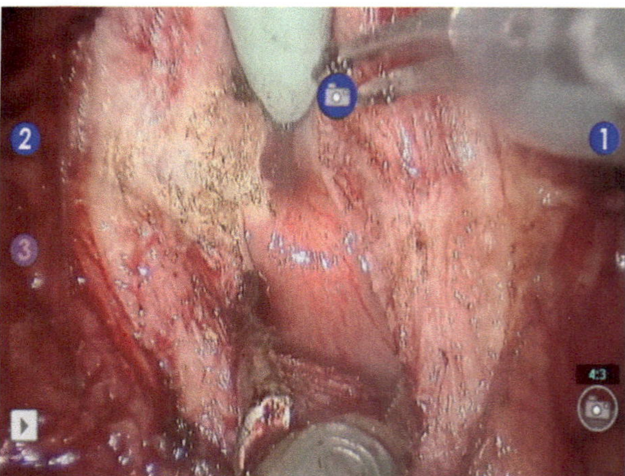

Fig. 7.5 Posterior bladder neck dissection – the precise junction between the prostate and the bladder is identified

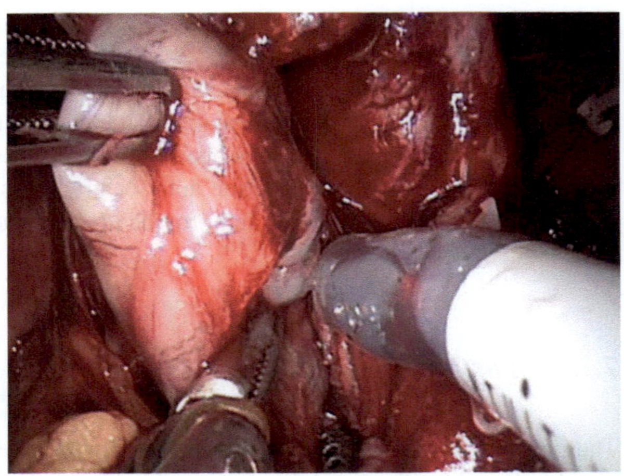

Fig. 7.6 Seminal vesicle dissection – the left vas deferens is retracted with the fourth arm. The medial avascular plane of the left seminal vesicle has been identified

vesicle (Fig. 7.6). Artery to the seminal vesicle is identified at this point and is clipped and cut. Once the artery is divided, the seminal vesicle is dissected and delivered out. Similarly, the contralateral vas and seminal vesicles are tackled.

7.3.7 Denonvilliers' Fascia and Posterior Dissection

The seminal vesicles are used for elevation of the prostate and identification of the posterior Denonvilliers' fascia. The Denonvilliers' fascia is incised at the base of the seminal vesicles. The correct plane is a clear pearly white plane which is avascular and separates easily when spread out with the scissor. The posterior space is widely dissected to completely release the prostate so as to facilitate its rotation during its nerve sparing (Fig. 7.7).

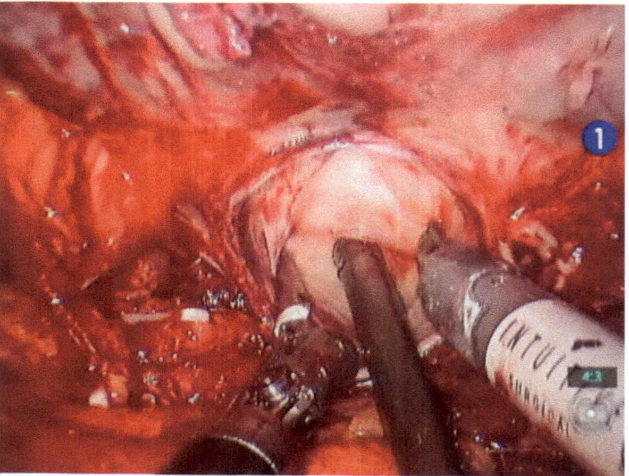

Fig. 7.7 Denonvilliers' fascia and posterior dissection

7.3.8 Nerve Sparing: Athermal Early Retrograde of the Neurovascular Bundle

We perform a retrograde nerve-sparing technique similar to the open approach. The neurovascular bundle is released prior to the prostatic pedicle. A thorough posterior dissection and adequate control of the dorsal venous complex are critical in decompressing large periprostatic veins that can cause significant bleeding during this step.

To facilitate release of neurovascular bundle, the prostate has to be rotated to the contralateral side. This rotation is done by the assistant on the left side and the fourth arm on the right side. With the prostate rotated medially, the lateral pelvic fascia and neurovascular bundle is identified and gently caressed away from the prostate with a mixture of sharp and blunt dissection. As the dissection is carried toward the apex of the prostate, an avascular plane between the prostate and the neurovascular bundle becomes apparent. The plane is continued posteriorly in a retrograde fashion between the neurovascular bundle and the prostatic fascia (interfascial nerve-sparing dissection). The prostatic pedicle is controlled with a Hem-o-lock clip placed away from the neurovascular bundle (Fig. 7.8). The NVB is then released distally to the level of the pelvic flow to prevent damage during apical dissection. The entire dissection of the neurovascular bundle has to be carried out athermally.

7.3.9 Apical Dissection

The landmarks are the ligated DVC, urethra, apex of the prostate, and NVB. It is essential to securely ligate the DVC to prevent bleeding, which may interfere with the apical dissection and division of the urethra under direct vision. Cold scissors

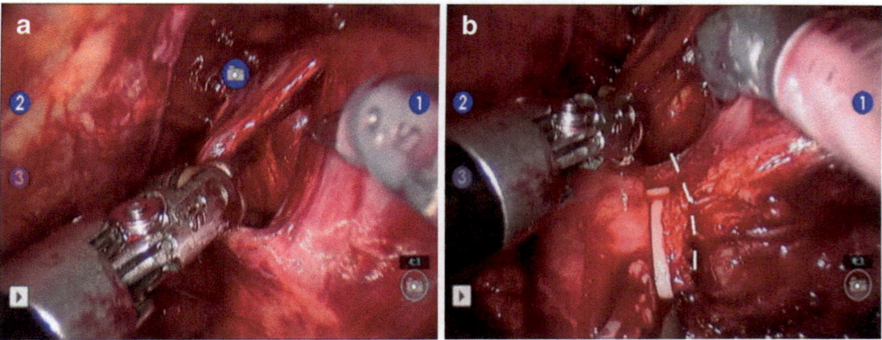

Fig. 7.8 Nerve sparing – "Athermal early retrograde release of the neurovascular bundle." (**a**) The avascular plane between the neurovascular bundle and prostatic fascia is developed. (**b**) The pedicle is controlled with a Hem-o-lock clip placed above the level of the already released bundle

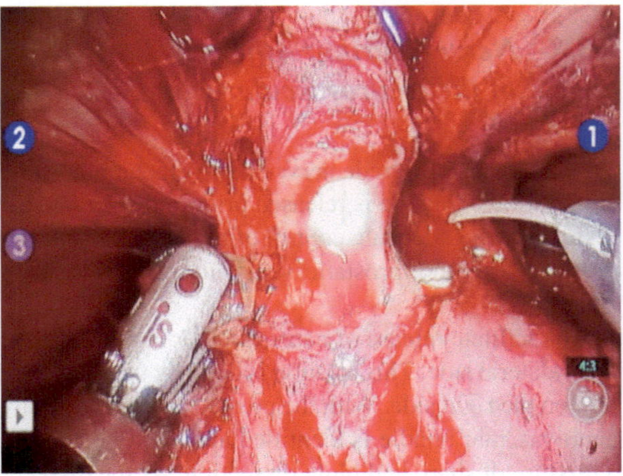

Fig. 7.9 Apical dissection

are used to divide the DVC, and a long urethral stump is developed. Complete dissection of the apex and urethra is facilitated by the robotic magnification. The urethra is then incised at the apex of the prostate under direct vision to completely liberate the prostate (Fig. 7.9).

7.3.10 Bladder Neck Reconstruction, Modified Posterior Reconstruction of the Rhabdosphincter, and Urethrovesical Anastomosis [15]

Before starting the bladder neck reconstruction, it is essential to check the position of ureteral orifices and their distance from the edge of the bladder neck. Bilateral plication over the lateral aspect of the bladder is then performed using

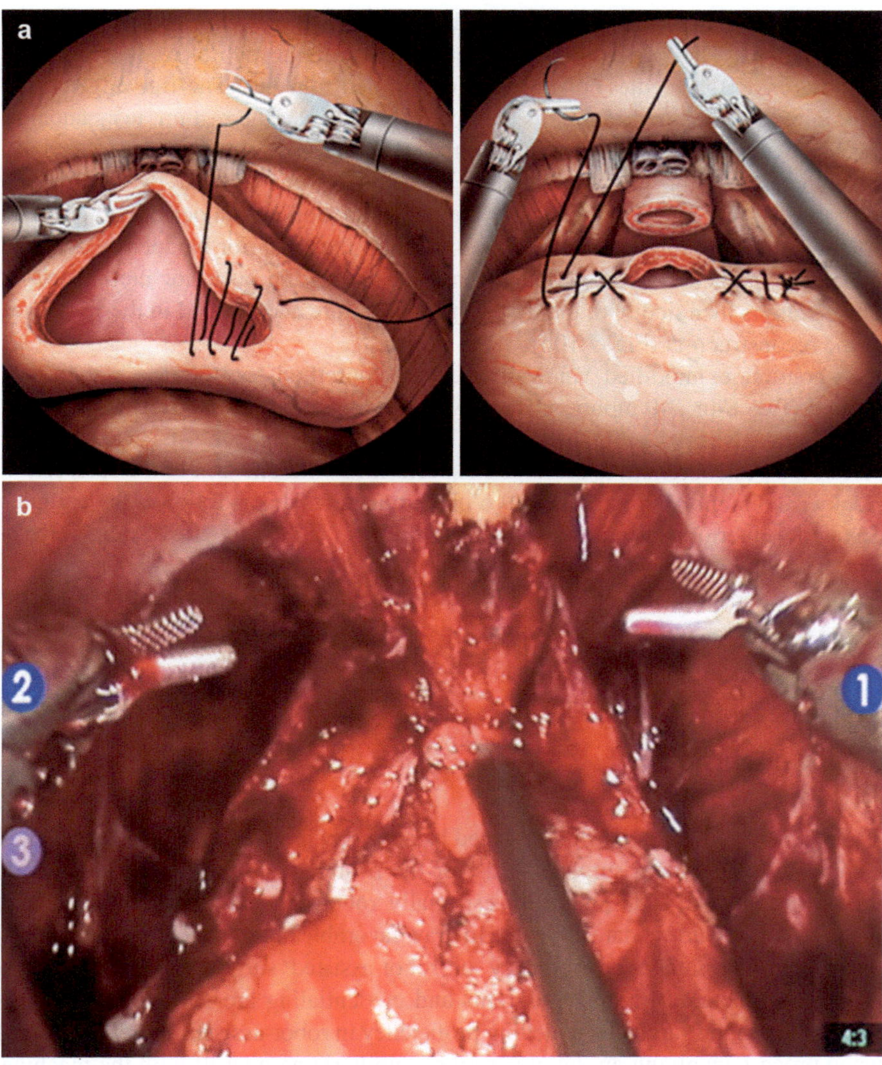

Fig. 7.10 Bladder neck reconstruction, modified posterior reconstruction of the rhabdosphincter, and vesicourethral anastomosis [13, 14]. (**a**) Bladder neck reconstruction. (**b**) Modified posterior reconstruction of the rabdosphincter – final aspect

sutures of 3-0 monocryl, with 6 in. length, in a RB-1 needle. The suture begins laterally and runs medially until the bladder neck size matches that of membranous urethra. The same suture subsequently runs laterally, back to the beginning of the suture in the lateral edge of the bladder neck; the suture is then tied (Fig. 7.10a).

Posterior reconstruction of the rhabdosphincter is performed prior to beginning the vesicourethral anastomosis. The principles are consistent with the two-layer reconstruction described previously by Rocco et al. with some technical modifications. The reconstruction is performed utilizing two 5-in. 3-0 monocryl sutures (on RB-1 needles) of different colors tied together. The free edge of the remaining Denonvilliers' fascia is identified anteriorly to the rectum, just caudal to the bladder neck. This edge is approximated to the posterior aspect of the rhabdosphincter and the posterior median raphe using one arm of the continuous monocryl suture. The second layer of the reconstruction is then performed with the other arm of the monocryl suture approximating the posterior bladder neck to the initial reconstructed layer of rhabdosphincter and to the posterior urethral edge. This suture is then tied with the first arm of the suture and utilized in the first layer of the reconstruction (Fig. 7.10b).

A continuous modified Van Velthoven vesicourethral anastomosis is then performed. Two 8-in. 3-0 monocryl sutures of different colors (on RB-1 needles) are tied together with 10 knots to provide a bolster for the anastomosis. The posterior part of the vesicourethral anastomosis is performed with one arm of the suture, in a clockwise direction, from the 5 to 9 o'clock position. This is followed by completion of the anterior anastomosis with the second arm of the suture in a counterclockwise fashion. An 18 Fr Foley catheter is then placed, and saline is irrigated to confirm watertight anastomosis. A JP drain is placed around the anastomosis, and all the trocars are removed under direct vision.

7.4 Conclusion

The recent introduction of robot-assisted laparoscopy has presented another level of technically challenging surgical skills for the postgraduate urologist. Robotics in urology is now in widespread use especially robot-assisted laparoscopic radical prostatectomy. Current data allows us to draw favorable initial conclusions about the reproducibility, safety, and efficacy of robot-assisted surgery in urology [16]. However, structured training programs and credentialing are still lacking for the upcoming robotic surgeon. Achieving proficiency in robot-assisted surgery is a multistep process involving an initial period of familiarizing oneself with the machine and mastering the basic skill set followed by advanced procedure-specific training with the help of a mentor. With better outcomes, advancements in instrumentation, and improvements in cost efficiency, robotics in surgery is bound to evolve and expand, and training and credentialing must keep pace with the developments.

References

1. Zorn KC, Gautam G, Shalhav AL, et al. Training, credentialing, proctoring and medicolegal risks of robotic urological surgery: recommendations of the society of urologic robotic surgeons. J Urol. 2009;182:1126–32.

2. Ahlering TE, Skarecky D, Lee D, et al. Successful transfer of open surgical skills to a laparoscopic environment using a robotic interface: initial experience with laparoscopic radical prostatectomy. J Urol. 2003;170:1738–41.
3. Vickers AJ, Bianco FJ, Serio AM, et al. The surgical learning curve for prostate cancer control after radical prostatectomy. JNCI. 2007;99:1171.
4. Link RE, Bhayani SB, Kavoussi LR. A prospective comparison of robotic and laparoscopic pyeloplasty. Ann Surg. 2006;243:486–91.
5. The Chamberlain Group Product Overview | Reproductive & Urological | Robotic [Internet]. [cited 2010 Aug 11];Available from: http://www.thecgroup.com/cat39/Reproductive-Urological/Robotic.html
6. Seixas-Mikelus SA, Kesavadas T, Srimathveeravalli G, et al. Face validation of a novel robotic surgical simulator. Urology. 2010;76:357–60.
7. Westwood JD, Hoffman HM, Mogel GT, et al. Medicine meets virtual reality 16: parallel, combinatorial, convergent : NextMed by design. IOS Press. (2008).
8. Nicholson Center for Surgical Advancement | Global Robotics Institute at Florida Hospital [Internet]. http://www.globalroboticsinstitute.com/en/urology-robotic-prostatectomy/nicholson-center
9. McDougall EM, Corica FA, Chou DS, et al. Short-term impact of a robot-assisted laparoscopic prostatectomy 'mini-residency' experience on postgraduate urologists' practice patterns. Int J Med Robot Comput Assist Surg. 2006;2:70–4.
10. Zorn KC, Wille MA, Thong AE, et al. Continued improvement of perioperative, pathological and continence outcomes during 700 robot-assisted radical prostatectomies. Can J Urol. 2009;16:4742.
11. Zorn KC, Orvieto MA, Gong EM, et al. Robotic radical prostatectomy learning curve of a fellowship-trained laparoscopic surgeon. J Endourol. 2007;21:441–7.
12. Rocco B, Lorusso A, Coelho RF, et al. Building a robotic program. Scand J Surg. 2009;98:72–5.
13. Hayat MJ, Howlader N, Reichman ME, et al. Cancer statistics, trends, and multiple primary cancer analyses from the Surveillance, Epidemiology, and End Results (SEER) Program. Oncologist. 2007;12:20–37.
14. Binder J, Kramer W. Robotically-assisted laparoscopic radical prostatectomy. BJU Int. 2001;87:408–10.
15. Lin VC, Coughlin G, Savamedi S, et al. Modified transverse plication for bladder neck reconstruction during robotic-assisted laparoscopic prostatectomy. BJU Int. 2009;104:878–81.
16. Ficarra V, Cavalleri S, Novara G, et al. Evidence from robot-assisted laparoscopic radical prostatectomy: a systematic review. Eur Urol. 2007;51:45–56.

Chapter 8
The Skills and Training Course of NOTES in Urology

Estevao A.R. Lima

Abstract Minimal invasiveness is ongoing and a novel development made possible by NOTES is to perform abdominal operations without any abdominal wall incisions. Several world NOTES consortiums have been established including a specialized Urology Working Group aiming to help develop urologic NOTES in a proper and safe way. The NOTES training is unique in that it crosses specialty shape, and most practitioners do not possess both the knowledge and skills to perform the procedures in their current form. Training with models allows mastering of basic techniques and realizing the difficulties of NOTES procedures.

Keywords Natural orifices translumenal endoscopic surgery • NOTES • Urology • Training course • Skill

8.1 Introduction

Urology could be considered one of the most "endoscopic" specialty among others. It focuses on procedures inside urinary cavities, and urologists have been aimed by a minimally invasive animus since ancient time. Indeed, the vesical endoscopy for diagnosis started in nineteenth century, and it progressed for therapy field of lower and upper urinary tract disease in twentieth century using transurethral approach without any scars [1]. Also in urology since the early 1990s, the shift toward less invasive procedures has made laparoscopy the first choice for the majority of procedure, overcoming progressively open laparotomy. It has become apparent that mini-

E.A.R. Lima, M.D., FEBU, Ph.D.
Department of Urology, Hospital of Braga,
Life and Health Sciences Research Institute (ICVS),
ICVS/3B's - PT Government Associate Laboratory,
School of Health Sciences, University of Minho Braga/Guimarães, Portugal
e-mail: estevaolima@ecsaude.uminho.pt

Y.H. Sun et al. (eds.), *The Training Courses of Urological Laparoscopy*,
DOI 10.1007/978-1-4471-2723-9_8, © Springer-Verlag London 2012

mally invasive surgery has been associated with faster recovery and earlier return to full activity. In addition, urologists would agree that the small incisions of laparoscopic surgery are associated with less pain and more cosmetic outcome than open laparotomy [2].

Simultaneously, other specialties as gastroenterology have changed progressively and dramatically over the last decades. Initially, endoscopic evaluation of the gastrointestinal tract was one of diagnosis and very limited therapy. Subsequently, endoscopic biopsy, hemorrhage control, and the snaring of polyps were a marked advance over previous methods of management, which often involved open exploration. Recently, endoscopists have expanded the indications for endoscopic therapeutic manipulation. There seems to be a convergence of the once separate ways of gastrointestinal endoscopy and surgery. However, the potential of flexible endoscopy to perform therapeutic procedures beyond the wall of the gastrointestinal tract was recognized in 1980 when the first percutaneous endoscopic gastrostomy (PEG) was described by Gauderer et al. [3]. More recently, Kozarek et al. showed that even pancreatic pseudocyst can be managed transgastrically [4].

In surgical field, the surgeon's desire went beyond the percutaneous access to abdominal cavity through the external wall with the dreaming intent of scarless surgery. With this purpose in 2004, the pioneers Kalloo et al. [5] from Boston, USA, described the transgastric access into the peritoneal cavity in porcine model, and Rao and Nageshwar Reddy [6] presented a video of the first human transgastric appendectomy at the Annual Conference of the Society of Gastrointestinal Endoscopy of India, giving the birth of a new paradigm, "the transluminal endoscopic surgery," nowadays, standardized as "natural orifice translumenal endoscopic surgery" (NOTES) [7].

NOTES is a rapidly evolving area of preclinical research, and several groups worldwide are developing this novel surgical approach together with industrial support. The concept of minimally invasive surgery, offering the advantages of minimal trauma to the abdominal wall and hence less postoperative pain, less wound complications, earlier patient mobilization, and shorter length of stay, is further expanded with NOTES. Peritoneal cavity is approached by using mouth, rectum, vagina, or urethra as ports of entry to the peritoneum instead of incisions on the abdominal wall. Performing abdominal operations without any abdominal wall incisions may offer all the advantages of minimal invasiveness and eliminate the complications associated with parietal wounds [7].

8.2 The History and the First's Experimental Studies in NOTES

Natural orifice surgery began in 1901 with Dimitri Ott who worked in Petrograd and described this technique as "ventroscopy" [8]. In this procedure, he used a speculum that was introduced through an incision in the posterior vaginal fornix. This transvaginal approach was forgotten till 1928 when Decker performed some culdoscopies [9]. In 2002, Gettman et al. described the first experimental application of natural orifice surgery when transvaginal nephrectomy was performed in the porcine model [10]. This procedure, indeed predated the acronym NOTES. He performed nephrectomy in five female pigs using a single 5-mm abdominal trocar; however, limitations related to the porcine model and instrumentation made the procedure cumbersome. Kalloo et al. reported the first natural orifice endoscopic surgery using a transgastric approach in a porcine model in which they orally introduced a flexible endoscope into the peritoneal cavity to perform peritoneoscopy and liver biopsies [5]. At procedure's end, researchers closed the gastric wall with endoscopic clips. In five experiments, all pigs recovered and gained weight.

Several studies have since used the transgastric port for intraperitoneal abdominal procedures, such as fallopian tube ligation, cholecystectomy, gastrojejunostomy, lymphadenectomy, oophorectomy, partial hysterectomy, splenectomy, diaphragmatic pacing, appendectomy, hernia repair, and pyloroplasty [11]. Following the initial enthusiasm, however, abdominal procedures through isolated transgastric routes raised limitations that jeopardized application in humans. Potential barriers to clinical practice included safe access to peritoneal cavity; gastric closure; infection prevention; spatial orientation; stable multitasking platform to obtain adequate anatomy exposure, organ retraction, secure grasping, and triangulation; difficulty in controlling the pneumoperitoneum; and management of iatrogenic intraperitoneal complications [7]. These limitations are primarily related with the nature of the gastroscope instruments (flexible and parallel), which made the surgeons lose some important principles from classical and laparoscopic surgery during transgastric procedures, such as: (i) absence of triangulation, (ii) poor retraction capability, and (iii) the necessity to work frequently in retroflexion with an inverted image.

Thus, Lima et al. hypothesized that the development of a lower abdominal port for introduction of rigid instruments would be a simple and easy way to overcome most of those limitations of the isolated transgastric port [12]. Using current urologic instruments, this group planned an atraumatic method to create a transvesical port. In a surviving experimental study, they demonstrated that the transvesical endoscopic approach to the peritoneal cavity was feasible and easy to create without any further complications in a porcine model, even when the vesicotomy is left opened just with a bladder catheter.

The transvesical port revealed properties to become an excellent access to the abdominal cavity. In fact, this access is naturally sterile. Anatomically, it is the most anterior lower abdominal port providing instrument access to the peritoneal cavity above the bowel loops. Moreover, it allowed the introduction of rigid instruments into the peritoneal cavity enhancing the possibility to retract structures in an easy way. The only disadvantage was due to the diameter of the urethra limiting specimen retrieval and the size of the instruments used by this approach.

Given the unexpected good results from first study using the transvesical route, Lima et al. tested the possibility to reach the thoracic cavity, after surpassing the diaphragm [13]. In this study, although the researchers had been able to perform only limited thoracoscopy and lung biopsies, it definitively extended the intervention field of NOTES from peritoneal to thoracic cavity as well.

Cholecystectomy has been considered the most challenging isolated transgastric approach. Using two endoscopes or a single endoscope conjugated with a transabdominal trocar, Park et al. and Swanstrom et al. experienced significant difficulties performing cholecystectomy using ShapeLock technology [14, 15]. Confirming the initial hypothesis that the transvesical approach would overcome some limitations of isolated transgastric access, Rolanda et al. demonstrated that adding the transvesical to the transgastric port provided the surgical team a better surgical triangulation and effective retraction [16]. In fact, with this strategy, this group reported for the first time the third-generation cholecystectomy by pure NOTES-combined accesses (transgastric and transvesical ports) launching the concept of combined or multiple ports for NOTES. More recently, Lima et al. used the same combined approach to perform nephrectomy [17].

Subsequently, other group from Harvard University developed the transcolonic access as concurrent with the transvesical approach. This study confirmed the benefits of a lower abdominal access, namely, the possibility to introduce rigid instruments and direct image from the upper abdominal organs, what pushed them to perform transcolonic cholecystectomy [18]. However, the transcolonic port retained many of the limitations previously described for the transgastric port, because it is not sterile, requiring a reliable and effective closure device that was not available even at this moment.

Given the ongoing difficulties in finding safe devices for endoscopic closure, several investigators tried to rediscover the transvaginal access (posterior colpotomy), which was being used for many years by the gynecologists to perform pelvic interventions. This access provided the same benefits as the transvesical and transcolonic accesses and revealed safe because it is easily closed without an endoscopic device since its closure is possible with current surgical stitches from the outside. In fact, the transvaginal port allows introduction of rigid instruments and organ retrieval even of large dimensions. These characteristics gave confidence to Zorron et al. from Rio de Janeiro in Brazil [19], Bessler et al. from New York in the United States [20], and Marescaux group from IRCAD, Strasbourg in France [21] to perform the first hybrid NOTES cholecystectomy using the combinations of transvaginal with transabdominal trocars in humans in 2007. In the same year, Clayman et al. reported transvaginal nephrectomy in porcine model performed using a purpose-built operating platform (TransPort Multi-lumen Operating Platform, USGI Medical, San Clemente, CA) [22]. The porcine kidney was mobilized exclusively through the vaginal port, and the renal hilum was controlled with an endovascular stapler placed through a 12-mm umbilical port.

More recently, using two 5-mm abdominal trocars and vaginal placement of an endoscope, Branco et al. described hybrid NOTES transvaginal nephrectomy to remove a nonfunctioning right kidney in a human [23]. This was the first clinical published application in the urological field of the hybrid concept indeed. Further minimizing the use of accessory transabdominal ports, in 2009, Kaouk and colleagues at the Cleveland Clinic successfully performed the world's first transvaginal NOTES nephrectomy on a 58-year-old woman who presented with an atrophic right kidney [24]. A single-port device was introduced transvaginally into the peritoneal cavity, and the instruments were placed across this port. There was no perioperative complication.

8.3 Working Groups in NOTES and Training

With these first descriptions of the NOTES procedures, there was a terrific debate about the potential benefits from transgastric access and the several challenges that it was causing regarding the several limitations that were being identified by the scarce groups that were testing mainly the transgastric port experimentally. In fact, there was a consensus that the transgastric access was not totally sterile and the difficulties in its endoscopic closure could be the cause of serious complications in abdominal surgery. Despite the aggressive criticisms from the most conservative surgeons and endoscopists, the possibility to perform scarless surgery nursed an increasing number of dreamers and believers in NOTES. Thus, in 2006, a joint effort from key persons from the American Society for Gastrointestinal Endoscopy (ASGE) and Society of American Gastrointestinal Endoscopic Surgeons (SAGES) organize the Natural Orifice Surgery Consortium for Assessment and Research (NOSCAR). This organization collected the preliminary data and summarized in a white paper the most important limitations and some potential strategies to overcome them. European researchers also formed the European Association of Transluminal Surgery (www.eats.fr), the EURO-NOTES Foundation (www.euro-notes.eu) to ease cooperation between the European Association for Endoscopic Surgery (EAES), and the European Society of Gastrointestinal Endoscopy (ESGE), and the New European Surgical Academy (NESA) (www.nesacademy.org) founded the Natural Orifice Surgery (NOS) working group, which is exploring another surgical route, the trans-douglas one. More recently, the Urology Working Group on NOTES of the Endourological Society (www.endourology.org) was created [25]. The initial objectives of this group was to: (i) increase awareness of NOTES in urology, (ii) provide an outlet to share discoveries related to urologic NOTES, (iii) guide scientific evaluation and implementation of urologic NOTES, (iv) facilitate learning opportunities with urologic NOTES, and (v) define nomenclature of urologic NOTES.

Indeed, the intention of the different world NOTES consortiums is the encouragement and stimulation of the safe introduction of NOTES techniques based on initial extensive experimental training followed by stepwise clinical application. Several studies have now demonstrated that NOTES can be performed, but there is a question of whether NOTES procedures can be performed safely. With the above in mind, the different working groups or consortiums strongly suggest a multidisciplinary team possessing advanced therapeutic endoscopic and advance laparoscopic skills to study NOTES before human investigation. Animal laboratory facilities to perform research and training should be available to the multidisciplinary team for exploration of NOTES techniques.

8.4 NOTES Training in Urology

With NOTES development, one must also address the issues of training. In fact, there needs to be increased access to courses and skills training for those interested in NOTES. The urologist involvement is paramount to the success of NOTES in urology. Postgraduate and hands-on courses will allow urologists to improve their skills and allow collaboration to help develop new technologies and direct future research in NOTES field. The future looks promising, although it will be some time before they will be used routinely.

Currently in Europe, NOTES hands-on course specific for urologists are offered by Life and Health Sciences Research Institute (ICVS), School of Health Sciences, University of Minho in Braga, Portugal (www.ecsaude.uminho.pt) (http://www.minimallyinvasiveurologicalweek.com) (Fig. 8.1). Other more general NOTES hands-on courses are also offered in other centers such as IRCAD in Strasburg, France (www.ircad.fr), "Centro de Cirugía Mínima Invasión" in Cáceres, Spain (www.ccmijesususon.com), and AIMS Advanced International Mini-invasive Surgery Academy in Milan, Italy (www.aimsacademy.org). Regularly, the University of Minho prepares updated and international environment hands-on courses centered in the participant requests and specially designed to provide expertise in the most cutting-edge techniques of NOTES. This academic center constituted with researchers with different scientific backgrounds and engineering that welcomes basic, translational, and clinical research projects that come up through a multidisciplinary way is aiming to contribute for a better understanding and resolution of surgical problems of NOTES. Moreover, helping to achieve this goal, this center have the collaboration of biomedical companies that supply the latest instruments, devices, and HD imaging hardware.

In this academic center, a variety of models have been developed to train urologists in NOTES skills within a structured curriculum. NOTES training is unique in that it crosses specialty shape (general surgery, urology, gynecology, gastroenterology), and most practitioners do not possess both the knowledge and skills to perform the procedures in their current form. The flexible endoscopy and instruments of gastroenterology used in NOTES are not familiar to most urologist and surgeon, while surgical technique and procedures are not familiar to most gastroenterologists. Moreover, the points of peritoneal access such as transvaginal, transcolonic, or transgastric are not well known to urologists and vice versa to other specialties, and the whole process becomes even more complex because the field is in constant evolution with advances in technology. This was the reason the leadership of both SAGES and ASGE has recommended that teams of physicians possessing both advanced endoscopic and laparoscopic skills perform NOTES procedures [7]. The combination of expertise in extralumenal and intralumenal pathology allowed carrying out NOTES procedures in a faster and safe way. Unfortunately, this consortium forgot the urologists and the urogenital tract.

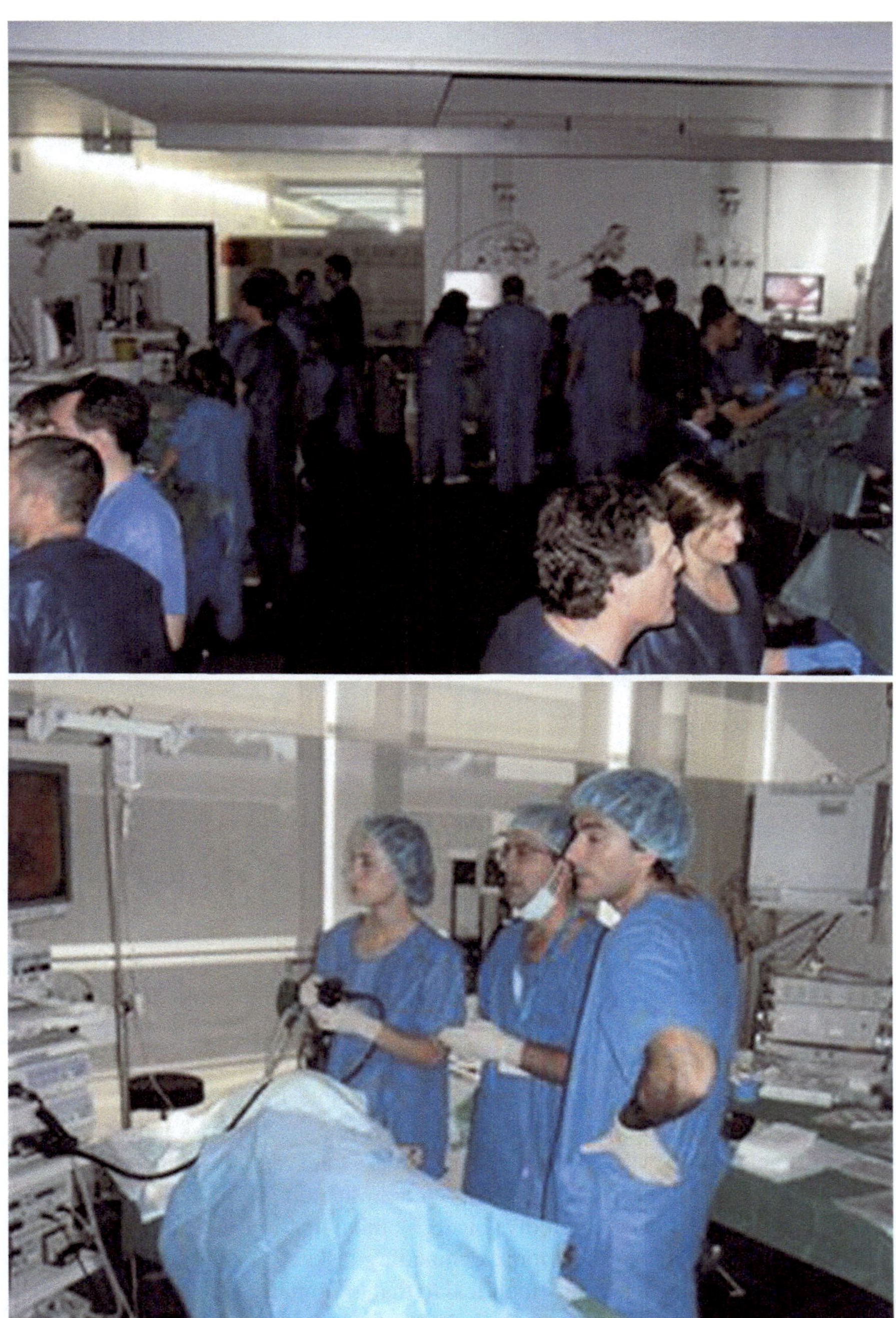

Fig. 8.1 Facilities and training of transgastric approach into the peritoneal cavity by urologists

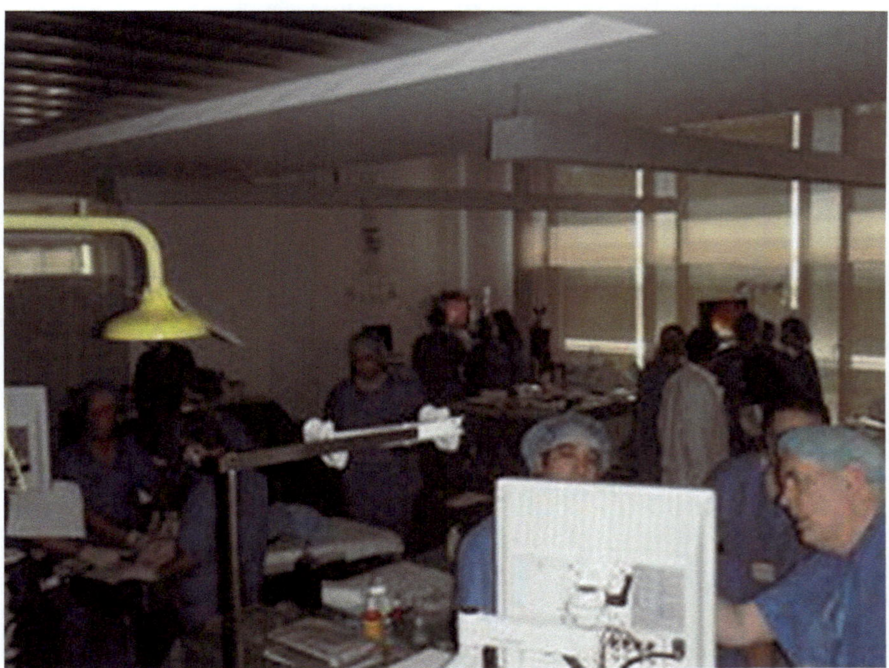

Fig. 8.1 (continued)

8.4.1 Models for Training in NOTES

Simulators and virtual reality have been argued to be effective in the acquisition of laparoscopic skills, and there may be a new role for simulators that are specifically designed for teaching translumenal surgery. The simulator provides a no-risk environment for the trainee to practice tasks and manage all possible complications. These features make the simulator a potential tool for training in NOTES in the future. However, animal models offer an alternative training system. The similarity of pig and human anatomy constitutes a valuable living model for learning NOTES skills. The urologists in training can practice the range of approaches into the peritoneal cavity (transgastric, transvesical, transvaginal, and transcolonic) and a wide variety of procedures such as cholecystectomy (Fig. 8.2), partial hepatectomy, splenectomy, nephrectomy (Fig. 8.3), tubal ligation, and varicocelectomy. The pig model covers easy and more demanding tasks. Considering that the anatomy of animals is not absolutely identical to that of humans, we have to accept that animal models are still far from ideal. Nevertheless, training with these models allows mastering of dissection techniques and realize the difficulties of NOTES procedures mainly related with the nature of the gastroscope instruments (flexible and parallel).

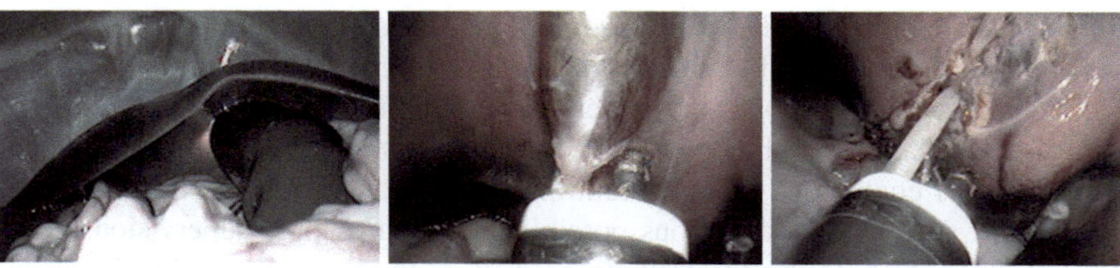

Fig. 8.2 Endoscopic view of gastroscope introduced into the peritoneal cavity by transgastric approach, starting the dissection of cystic channel, dissection of gallbladder

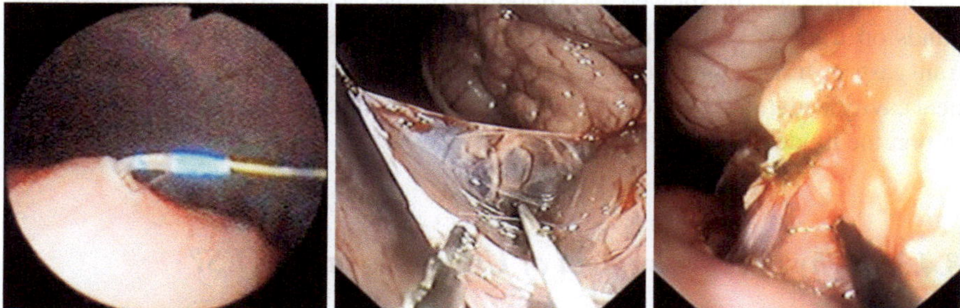

Fig. 8.3 Creation of gastrostomy, dissection of parietal peritoneum for hilar approach, renal artery ligated, and dissection of renal vein

8.4.2 NOTES Training Program

The Minho University NOTES course suggested a training program, during which each participant has a half day of theory teaching module and two days of hands-on module. During the teaching module, each trainee will: (i) understand rationale and challenges of NOTES; (ii) learn how to set up a research lab for NOTES procedure; (iii) summarize available instruments, operative platforms, and access techniques in NOTES; (iv) review all current NOTES and hybrid NOTES experience on humans and identify future human applications; and (v) understand the importance of hybrid techniques and patient selection.

The hands-on training module is carrying out on a swine model using animals with median weight of 30 kg. General anesthesia is performed in all cases. The training program supported by a multidisciplinary faculty (urologist, general surgeon, gastroenterologist) is designed to include: (i) transgastric approach of the peritoneal cavity with tubal ligation, varicocelectomy, and cholecystectomy; (ii) transvesical approach of the peritoneal cavity with combined transvesical and transgastric or hybrid nephrectomy; (iii) transvaginal approach with hybrid nephrectomy; and (iv) possibility of conduct experiment in transcolonic approach into the peritoneal cavity. Another important step before the initiation of procedures is the safe creation of viscerotomies (e.g., penetration of the anterior gastric wall with a flexible needle knife in order to be able to advance the scope from the gastric lumen outside into the peritoneal cavity) without damaging neighboring organs. This is facilitated by a laparoscopic control view for safety purposes with an assisting trocar usually placed periumbilically. Moreover, the assisting trocar fulfills additional two tasks: (i) continuous pressure-controlled pneumoperitoneum via the laparoscopic port and (ii) the continuous possibility of laparoscopic supervision of the NOTES procedure during the training as well as the possibility of assisting by grasping retraction or application of clips and stapling. Then, the trainee performed all steps of the program supported by one assisting nurse for handing of the necessary instruments. Tips and tricks to overcome the learning curve and initial technical difficulties will be showed and supported by the faculty. At the conclusion of the hands-on training session of NOTES, the participants should be able to perform transgastric, transcolonic, transvaginal, and transvesical approaches to the peritoneal cavity with tubal ligation, cholecystectomy, nephrectomy, and varicocelectomy in porcine model.

8.4.3 *Why the Involvement of Urologists in NOTES?*

NOTES may present a tremendous challenge for urologists in terms of technical demands. It may also involve multidisciplinary teams to deal with nonurologic clinical situations, considering the simplicity of accessing and viewing the upper abdominal organs via the transvesical port [26] (Fig. 8.4).

In animal and human settings, the transvesical port enables feasible and useful peritoneoscopy of all intra-abdominal viscera, mainly the upper abdominal organs [27]. Further, the transvesical port is gaining a place in NOTES as a unique port associated with the transgastric port. Rolanda et al. and Lima et al. demonstrated the utility of a combined transgastric and transvesical approach, performing a reliable, feasible, exclusive NOTES cholecystectomy and nephrectomy [16, 17]. These

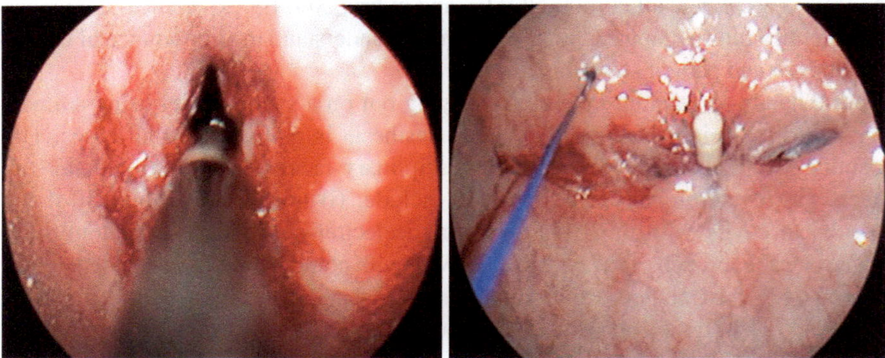

Fig. 8.4 Transvesical approach into the peritoneal cavity with the creation of vesicotomy in the bladder dome, ending endoscopic suture of the vesicotomy closure (second pair of T-tags applied)

studies emphasized the transvesical port's ability to overcome limitations of procedures performed exclusively through a transgastric port.

Although possibly difficult to accept clinically, the transvesical port provides exceptional access to the upper abdominal organs and may enable a transdiaphragmatic endoscopic approach to the thoracic cavity in a long-term survival study in a porcine model [13]. Most of these studies are preliminary and only represent the birth of NOTES in urology; however, they demonstrate a need for new instruments and further research that provides evidence that experimental success may advantageously translate to clinical practice in humans.

8.5 Conclusions

In many areas of medicine, divisions between specialties are blurring. For example, stent placement for carotid stenosis is now performed by neuroradiologists, interventional radiologists, vascular surgeons, and cardiologists. Similar reports commonly occur in other clinical areas. Currently, NOTES procedures and research are primarily performed by gastroenterologists and surgeons. However, because the mouth and colon are not the only access points, urologists and gynecologists have approached the peritoneum through the bladder and vagina. Further, NOTES has enabled transvaginal nephrectomy, peritoneoscopy, and thoracoscopy using a transvesical approach, and cholecystectomy and nephrectomy using a combined transvesical and transgastric approach. These procedures have mostly been performed in animal models, but human application is pending.

Urologists have been encouraged in this developing field to meet an especially great demand should NOTES develop as some investigators have proposed. Clinicians embarking on human studies need to be trained sufficiently in the laboratory and with animal models to minimize and standardize NOTES complications.

In the future, the design of residency and fellowship programs may shift toward developing urologists who are facile in achieving the peritoneal cavity using different peritoneal accesses (mouth, bladder, vagina, and colon). Until then, the development of validated training and testing programs is imperative before the wide-scale performance of NOTES procedures.

References

1. Gettman MT, Box G, Averch T, et al. Consensus statement on natural orifice transluminal endoscopic surgery and single-incision laparoscopic surgery: heralding a new era in urology? Eur Urol. 2008;53:1117–20.
2. Harrell AG, Heniford T. Minimally invasive abdominal surgery: lux et veritas past, present, and future. Am J Surg. 2005;190:239–43.
3. Gauderer MW, Ponsky JL, Izant Jr RJ. Gastrostomy without laparotomy: a percutaneous endoscopic technique. J Pediatr Surg. 1980;15:872–5.

4. Kozarek RA, Brayko CM, Harlan J. Endoscopic drainage of pancreatic pseudocysts. Gastrointest Endosc. 1985;31:322–7.
5. Kalloo AN, Singh VK, Jagannath SB. Flexible transgastric peritoneoscopy: a novel approach to diagnostic and therapeutic interventions in the peritoneal cavity. Gastrointest Endosc. 2004;60:114–7.
6. Reddy N, Rao P. Per oral transgastric endoscopic appendectomy in human. In: Abstract presented at 45th annual conference of the Society of Gastrointestinal Endoscopy of India; Jaipur, 2004.
7. Rattner D, Kalloo A. ASGE/SAGES Working Group on Natural Orifice transluminal endoscopic surgery SAGES/ASGE Working Group on NOTES. Surg Endosc. 2006;20:329–33.
8. Ott DO. Ventroscopic illumination of the abdominal cavity in pregnancy. Z Akus Zhenskikl Bolezn. 1901;15:7–8.
9. Decker A. Culdoscopy: a method for visual diagnosis of gynecologic disease. Clin Symp. 1952;6:201–10.
10. Gettman MT, Lotan Y, Napper CA, et al. Transvaginal laparoscopic nephrectomy: development and feasibility in the porcine model. Urology. 2002;59:446–50.
11. Lima E, Rolanda C, Correia-Pinto J. NOTES performed using multiple ports of entry: current experience and potential implications for urologic applications. J Endourol. 2009;23:759–64.
12. Lima E, Rolanda C, Pêgo JM, et al. Transvesical endoscopic peritoneoscopy: a novel 5 mm-Port for intra-abdominal scarless surgery. J Urol. 2006;176:802–5.
13. Lima E, Henriques-Coelho T, Rolanda C, et al. Transvesical thoracoscopy: a natural orifice transluminal endoscopic approach for thoracic surgery. Surg Endosc. 2007;21:854–8.
14. Park PO, Bergstrom M, Ikeda K, et al. Experimental studies of transgastric gallbladder surgery: cholecystectomy and cholecystogastric anastomosis (videos). Gastrointest Endosc. 2005;61:601–6.
15. Swanstrom LL, Kozarek R, Pasricha PJ, et al. Development of a new access device for transgastric surgery. J Gastrointest Surg. 2005;9:1129–37.
16. Rolanda C, Lima E, Pêgo JM, et al. Third generation cholecystectomy by natural orifices: transgastric and transvesical combined approach. Gastrointest Endosc. 2007;65:111–7.
17. Lima E, Rolanda C, Pêgo JM, et al. Third-generation nephrectomy by natural orifice transluminal endoscopic surgery. J Urol. 2007;178:2648–54.
18. Pai RD, Fong DG, Bundga ME, et al. Transcolonic endoscopic cholecystectomy: a NOTES survival study in a porcine model (with video. Gastrointest Endosc. 2006;64:428–34.
19. Zorron R, Maggioni LC, Pombo L, et al. NOTES transvaginal cholecystectomy: preliminary clinical application. Surg Endosc. 2008;22:542–7.
20. Bessler M, Stevens PD, Milone L, et al. Transvaginal laparoscopically assisted endoscopic cholecystectomy: a hybrid approach to natural orifice surgery. Gastrointest Endosc. 2007;66:1243–5.
21. Marescaux J, Dallemagne B, Perretta S, et al. Surgery without scars: report of transluminal cholecystectomy in a human being. Arch Surg. 2007;142:823–6.
22. Clayman RV, Box GN, Abraham JB, et al. Rapid communication: transvaginal single-port NOTES nephrectomy: initial laboratory experience. J Endourol. 2007;21:640–4.
23. Branco AW, Filho AJ, Kondo W, et al. Hybrid transvaginal nephrectomy. Eur Urol. 2007;53:1290–4.
24. Kaouk JH, Haber GP, Goel RK, et al. Pure natural orifice translumenal endoscopic surgery (NOTES) transvaginal nephrectomy. Eur Urol. 2010;57(4):723–6.
25. Box G, Averch T, Cadeddu J, et al. Nomenclature of natural orifice translumenal endoscopic surgery (NOTES) and laparoendoscopic single-site surgery (LESS) procedures in urology. J Endourol. 2008;22:2575–81.
26. Lima E, Rolanda C, Osório L, et al. Endoscopic closure of transmural bladder wall perforations. Eur Urol. 2009;56:151–7.
27. Gettman MT, Blute ML. Transvesical peritoneoscopy: initial clinical evaluation of the bladder as a portal for natural orifice translumenal endoscopic surgery. Mayo Clin Proc. 2007;82:843–5.

Chapter 9
The Tips and Tricks of the Suture in Urologic Laparoscopy

Eugen Yuhui Wang

Abstract The basic principles in suturing and knotting should be learned and followed before attempting to study more complex endolaparoscopic knotting and suturing techniques. Laparoscopic square knots are to be as secure as open square knots, and there is no substantive difference in the security of laparoscopic intracorporeally and extracorporeally tied knots. The perfect needle holder should be ergonomic, light, have a hard needle grip and at the same time easy to change needle positioning. The optimal angle between the tip of the needle holder and the needle should be around 90°. For anastomosis suturing, optimal distance between trocars is 12 cm. Optimal angle between needle holders is <45°. Optimal angle between needle holders and anastomosis is 55°. Suturing in the right lateral positions of the camera is much easier for right-handed surgeons.

Keywords Urology • Laparoscopy • Surgery • Suture • Tips • Tricks

9.1 Introduction

Although laparoscopy has been applied in practice by urologists for nearly two decades [1], the penetration of urologic laparoscopy in the world remains less than ideal. Laparoscopy (multi- and/or single incision) requires a skill set fundamentally different from traditional open surgery. Since robotic-assisted laparoscopic surgery

E.Y. Wang, M.D., Ph.D., FEBU
Department of Urology, Clinic for Urology and Andrology,
Eskilstuna/Stockholm, Sweden

Centre for Clinical Research Sörmland, Uppsala University,
Kungsgata 41, 633 40, Eskilstuna, Sweden
e-mail: info@drwang.se

Y.H. Sun et al. (eds.), *The Training Courses of Urological Laparoscopy*,
DOI 10.1007/978-1-4471-2723-9_9, © Springer-Verlag London 2012

in urology has quickly developed, some specialists consider that robotics represents "enabling technology" whereby those without adequate training in laparoscopy would be able to perform complex minimally invasive procedures [2–4]. However, it is undisputed that essential laparoscopic techniques, such as endolaparoscopic suturing and knotting, are supplanted by robotics for most conditions and procedures [5]. Training in laparoscopy as a modality will continue to have merit in educational curricula [6]. Intracorporeal knot, suturing, and anastomosis are still large hidden challenges due to spatial limitation and difficulty of exposure, together with a fixed trocar position and long and rigid instrument. In the literature, there are only a few reports on the standardization of laparoscopic intracorporeal suturing and knotting techniques [7, 8]. Therefore, the actual surgical technique needs to be analyzed and optimized. This includes not only sufficient standardization of intracorporeal and extracorporeal suturing and knotting techniques and optimizing of the suture materials and instruments but also the evaluation of further important "geometric" factors of endoscope reconstruction, such as the optimal distances between the working trocars, length of the instruments, and angles between the instruments and the object [9, 10]. In this chapter, we will introduce some tips and tricks of endolaparoscopic suturing and knotting techniques which attempt to get optimal access in more complex laparo- and retroperitoneoscopic or robotic procedures, as well as effort to develop standards for the best possible approach under these limited conditions.

9.2 Some Basic Technique Principles in Suturing and Knotting

There are some basic technique principles from needle grasping, suturing, to knotting. At the very beginning, we would like to point out these basic technique principles, which should be followed in almost every surgical procedure in open, laparoscopic, as well as robotic surgery:

- Needle grasped at "sweet spot" by dominant hand with or without "pirouette."
- Abduction to approach surface with needle at 90° (perpendicular to tissue).
- Needle position used in "smiley face up" with "toe in."
- Needle tip clearance adequate for grasping on other side of tissue.
- Suture pulled until tail of appropriate length (needle toward the sky).
- Penetration of tissue followed by rotation with support of tissue by other instrument.
- This applies to monofilament as well as multifilament sutures.
- Avoid damaging the suture with instruments.
- Use the simplest knot for the material.
- The knot must be firm to prevent slipping.
- The knot must be as small as possible.
- Ends should be cut as short as possible without creating knot instability.
- Excessive tension may break sutures and cut tissue.

- Approximate, do not strangulate.
- Avoiding excessive tension allows use of finer sutures.
- Ideally, the two ends of the suture should be pulled in opposite directions with equal tension.
- The surgeon should not hesitate to change stance or position in relation to the patient to place a knot securely and flat.
- Extra throws do not add to strength of a properly tied knot, only to its bulk.

Only when you have finished studying and followed these principles can you continue to study more different knotting and suturing techniques.

9.3 Different Knotting Techniques

Here within we would like to present different knotting techniques step by step from extra- to intracorporeal procedures.

9.3.1 Endoligature with Extracorporeal Knotting

9.3.1.1 Roeder Slipknot (Fig. 9.1a–h)

1. Make one short limb (the post) and one long limb (the loop).
2. Throw the loop, then around the post.
3. Next, throw the loop around both limbs.
4. Throw the loop only around the post limb.
5. Pass the tail of the loop limb between the second and third loop.
6. The knot is tensioned and pushed into the joint with a knot pusher on the post limb.
7. The knot is secured with a series of half hitches, thrown in alternate directions [11].

In practice, you can make Roeder knot extracorporeally, as shown in Fig. 9.2a–d.

9.3.1.2 Jamming Anchor Knot: A Continuous Suture Line Starting Knot (Figs. 9.3a–d and 9.4a–d)

1. Start with 25 cm or 10 in. of suture attached to a needle.
2. Extracorporeally, make the Dundee jamming knot from the distal 5 cm or 2 in. of suture.

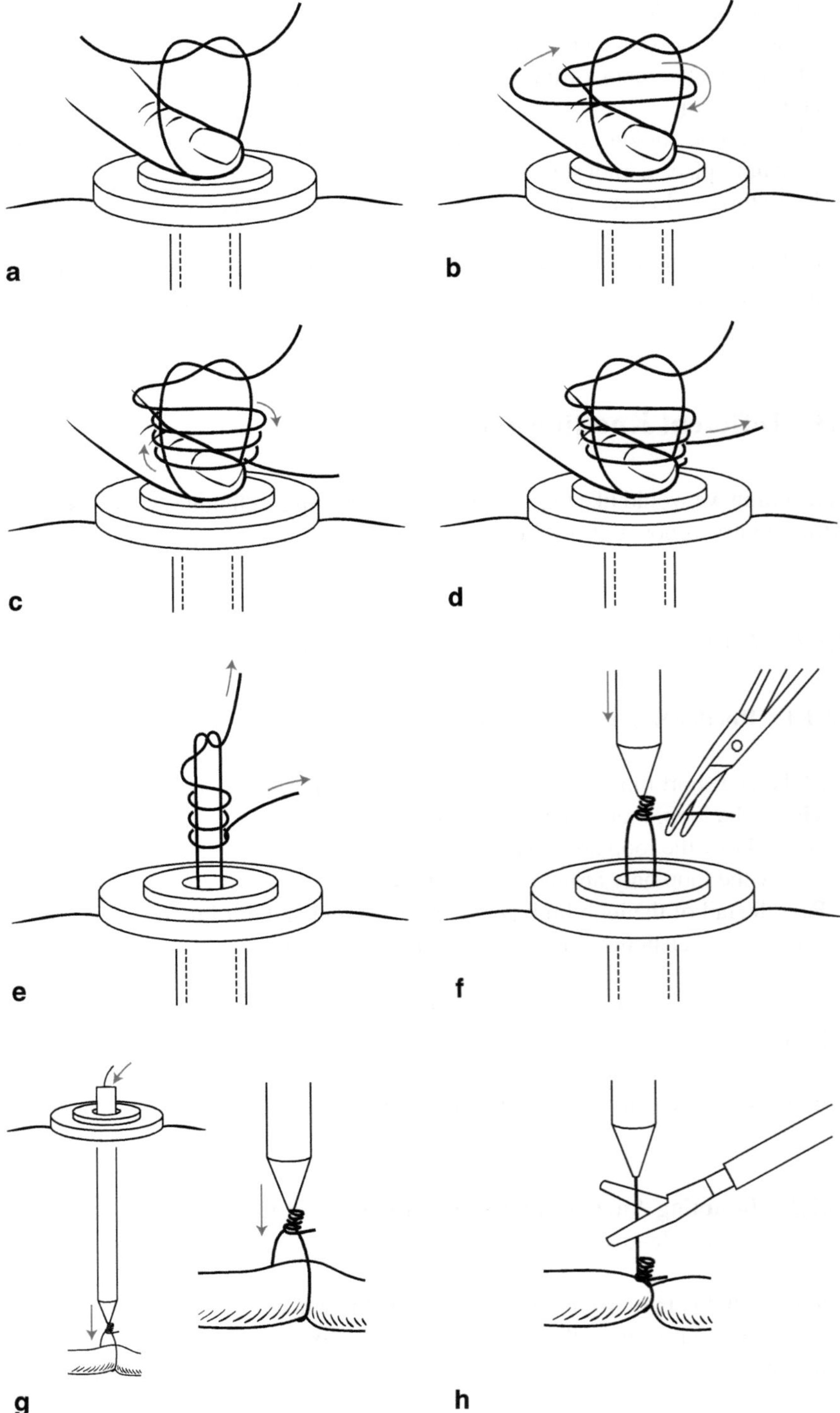

Fig. 9.1 (**a**–**h**) Roeder slipknot

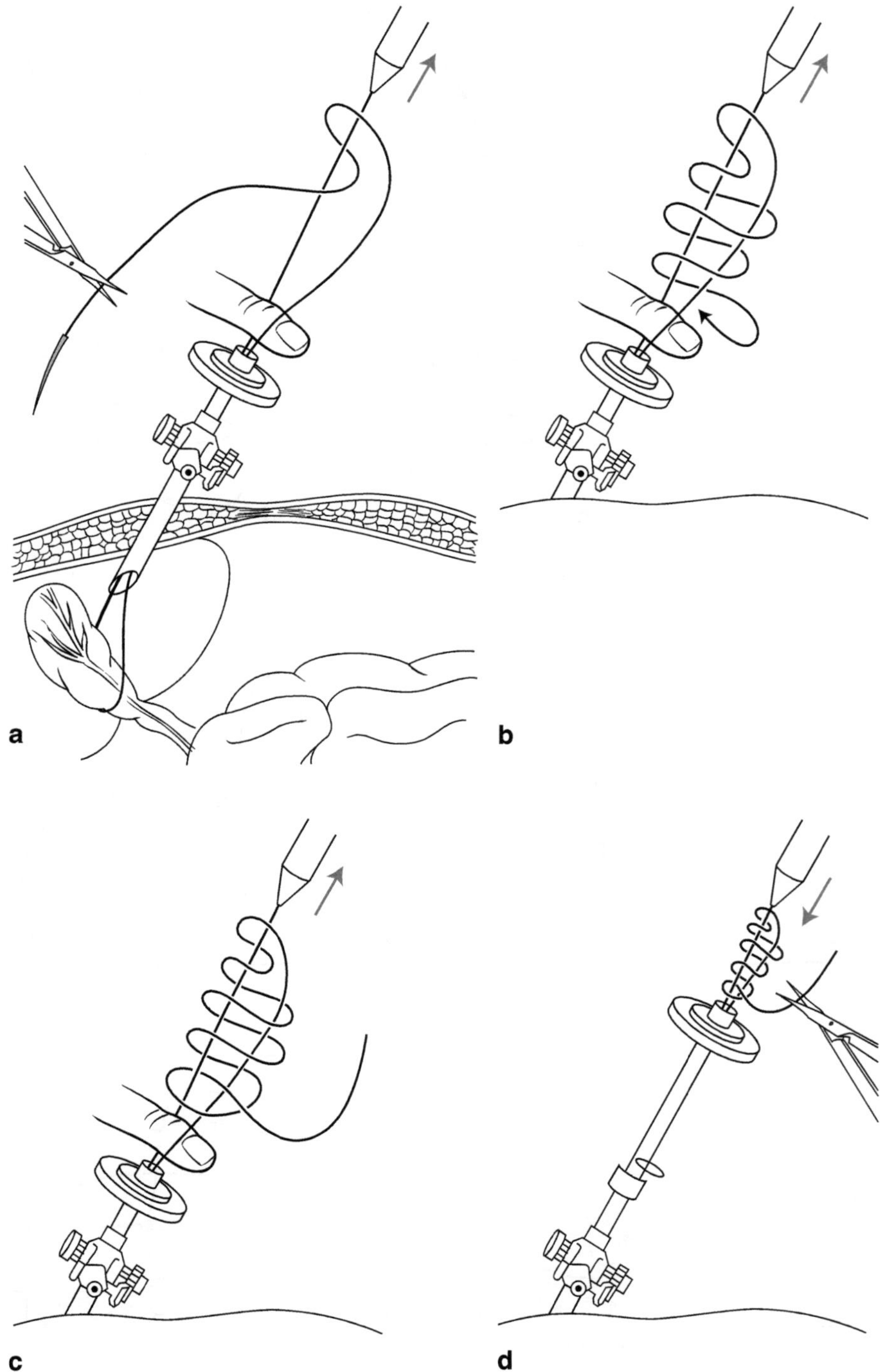

Fig. 9.2 (**a**–**d**) Make a Roeder knot extracorporeally

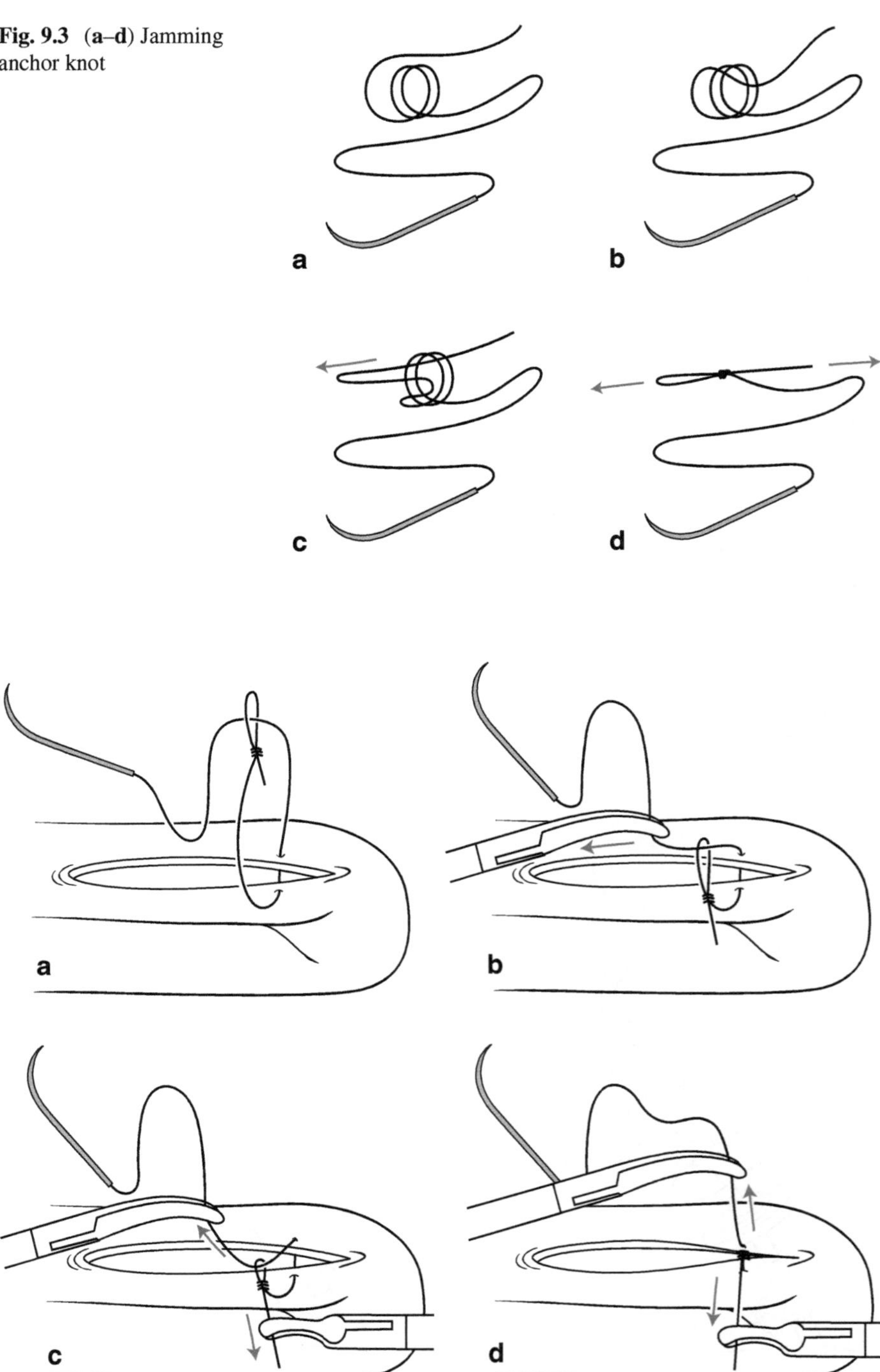

Fig. 9.3 (**a–d**) Jamming anchor knot

Fig. 9.4 (**a–d**) A continuous suture line starting knot – jamming anchor knot

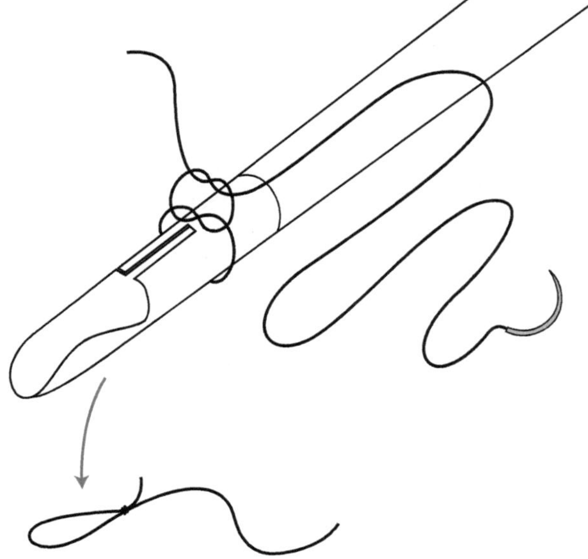

Fig. 9.5 An end knot loop similar to jamming anchor knot

3. Bring the suture and attached needle into the abdomen.
4. Place the first suture across both sides of the tissue.
5. Bring the suture and attached needle through the loop of the Dundee jamming knot.

There is an alternate method of forming end knot loop similar to jamming anchor knot, which is practically used often (Fig. 9.5).

9.3.1.3 Heaving Line Knot: A Continuous Suture Starting Knot (Fig. 9.6)

1. Start with 25 cm or 10 in. of suture attached to a needle.
2. Extracorporeally, make the heaving line knot from the distal 5 cm or 2 in. of suture.
3. You may apply a clip just proximal to the knot (toward the needle) for added security.
4. Bring the suture and attached needle into the abdomen.
5. The heaving line knot forms an adequate end knot by itself.

Intracorporeally, you can follow to make a heaving line knot. Fig. 9.7a–c.

9.3.1.4 Meltzer Knot (Modified Roeder Knot) (Fig. 9.8a–d)

1. Requires 1.5 m or 150 cm or 60 in. of suture.
2. Use braided suture material, such as Dacron or Lactomer.

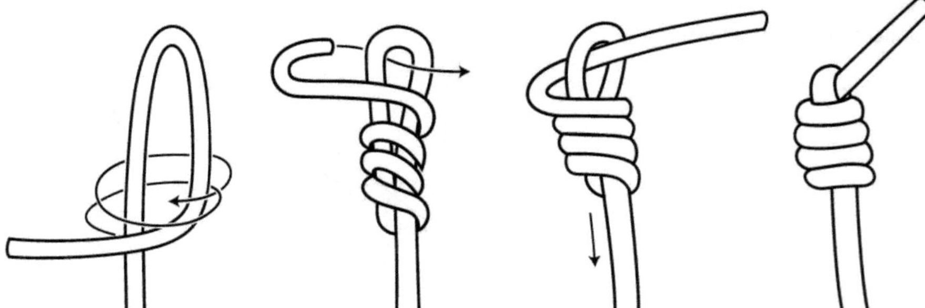

Fig. 9.6 A continuous suture starting knot – heaving line knot

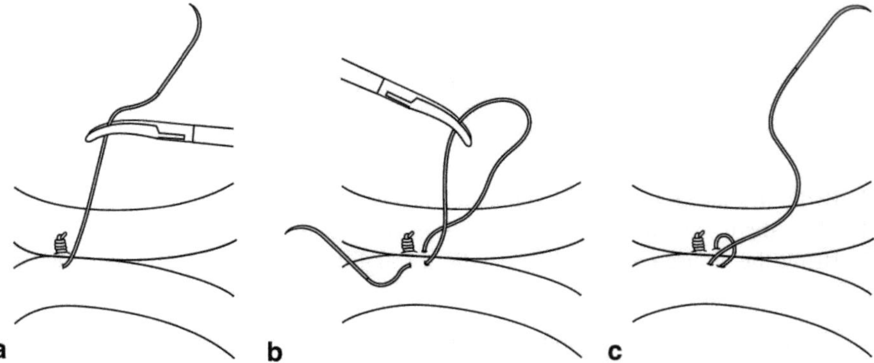

Fig. 9.7 (**a**) When the heaving line stopper knot is used, the suture – after needle passage through the two organs – is simply pulled until the stopper knot abuts on one side of the intended anastomosis. (**b**, **c**) As the suture is held taut by the assistant, a second needle passage through the two organs close to the first is made (**a**) and the suture locked (**b**)

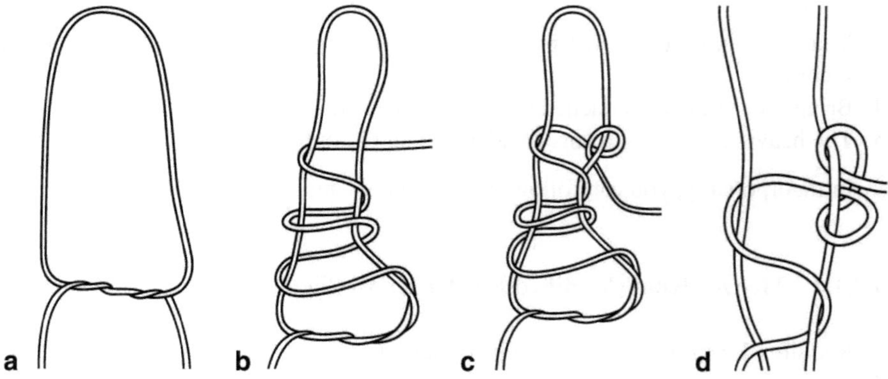

Fig. 9.8 (**a**–**d**) Meltzer knot (modified Roeder knot)

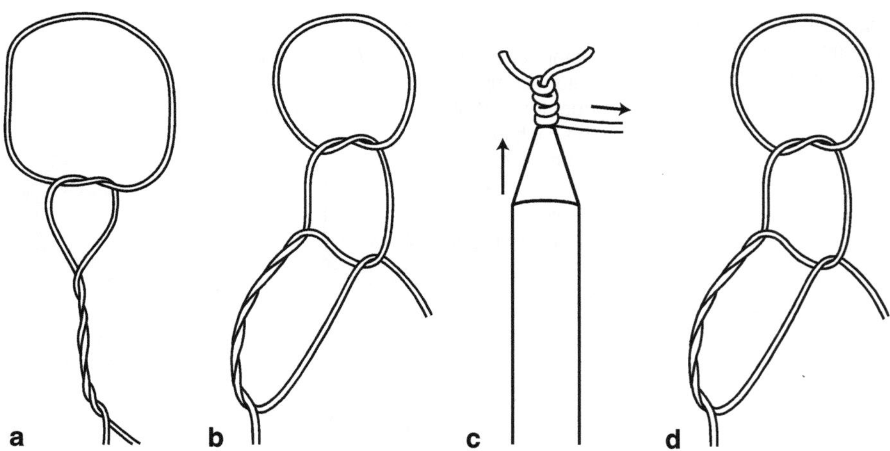

Fig. 9.9 (**a–d**) Tayside knot

3. Meltzer knot is reasonably secure with monofilament polydioxanone.
4. Slide the knot down and do not pull up on it like a lasso (used by American cowboys to rope calves). Pulling up on the Meltzer knot to snug it would saw through and tear the tissue.

9.3.1.5 Tayside Knot (Fig. 9.9a–d)

1. More secure than the Roeder knot, but slides down less easily.
2. Requires 1.5 m or 150 cm or 60 in. of suture.
3. Slide the knot down and do not pull up on it like a lasso (used by American cowboys to rope calves).
4. Pulling up on the Tayside knot to snug it would saw through and tear the tissue.
5. After you slide the knot down, pull on the tail or short end to secure the knot [12].

9.3.2 Endoligature with Intracorporeal Knotting Aberdeen Knot (Fig. 9.10a–d)

1. A loop or bight is formed in the suture (A) and passed under the bar. In surgery, the loop is taken as the last bight of the suture line.
2. A further loop or bight (B) is formed in the working end and passed through the loop A.
3. The bight B has been passed through A. This is called a throw. This step can be repeated any number of times to give varying numbers of throws.
4. To finish the knot, the end of the suture, C, is then passed through the new loop formed by the previous bight, B. This is called "one turn."

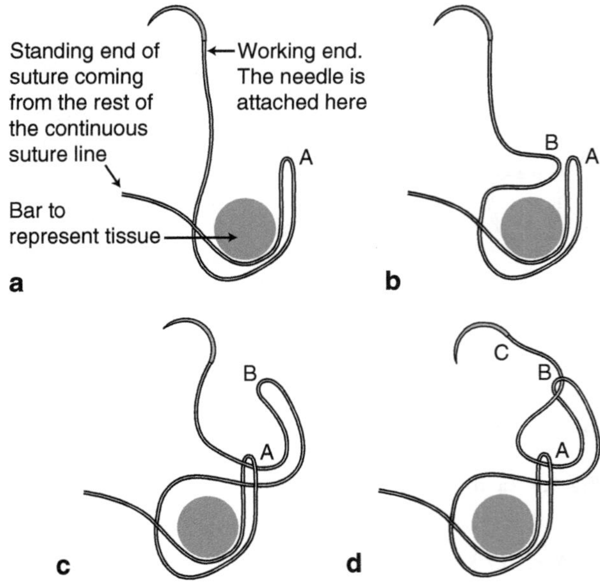

Fig. 9.10 (**a–d**) Endoligature with intracorporeal knotting Aberdeen Knot13

9.3.3 Intracorporeally, You Can Follow as Fig. 9.11a–h

9.3.4 Slipping Square Knot (Fig. 9.12a–h)

1. Use to snug down a square knot when the first throw comes loose. You can also use this technique to secure a surgeon's knot if the first throw comes loose.
2. Place a second throw and leave it loose.
3. Pull the long end of the suture toward you and the tail away from you. This converts the knot to two eyelets which will slip to snug the knot.
4. After the knot is snug, set it by pulling both ends laterally.

9.3.5 Intracorporeally, You Can Do Square/Slipknot as Fig. 9.13a–f

9.3.6 Sometimes You Can Make Square Knot as a Slipknot (Fig. 9.14a–d)

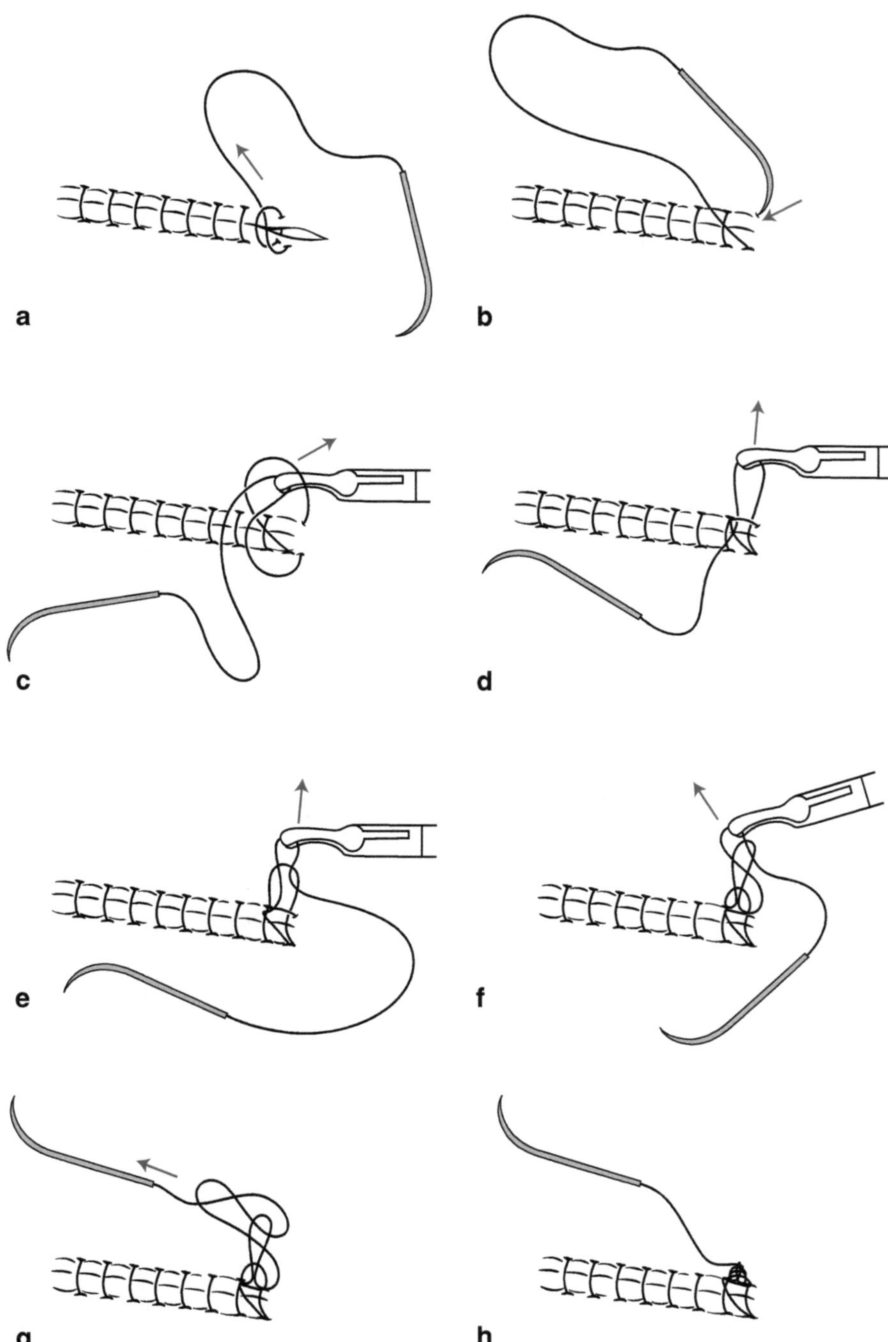

Fig. 9.11 (**a–h**) Aberdeen knot extracorporeally

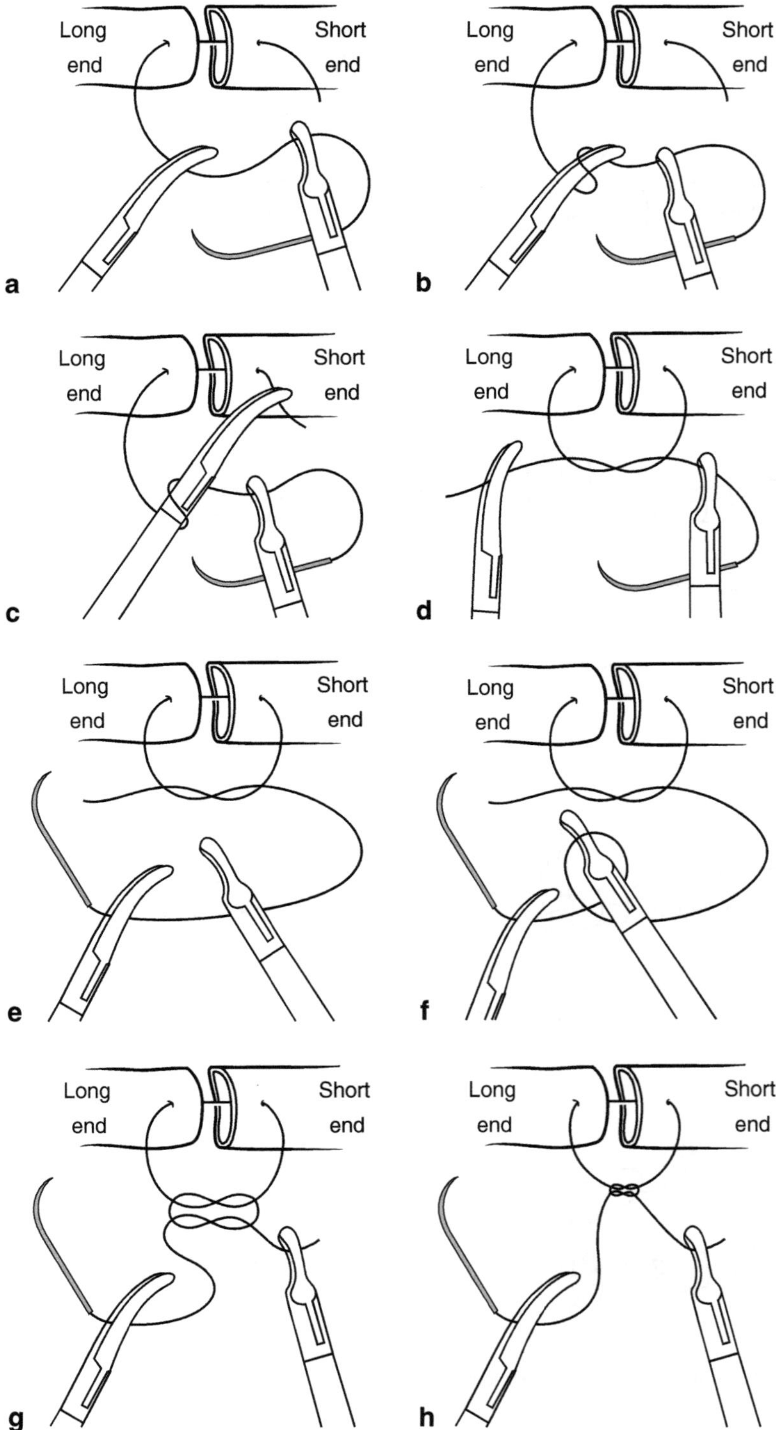

Fig. 9.12 (**a–h**) Slipping square knot [13]

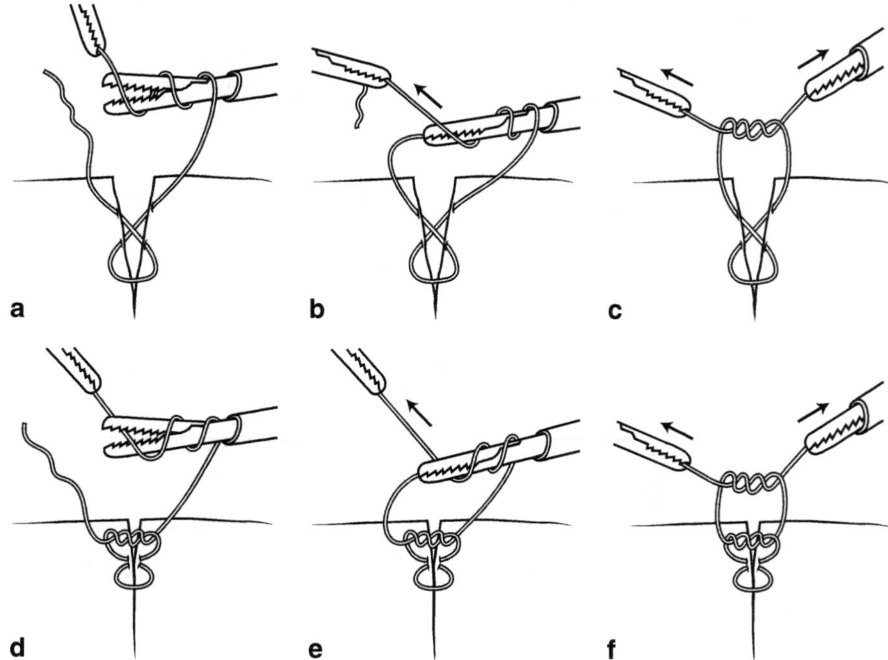

Fig. 9.13 (**a–f**) Square/slipknot with needle holder

9.4 Laparoscopic Knot Material and Security

The security of several types of laparoscopic knots and varying suture materials was tested in an attempt to improve suture and knot selection for advanced laparoscopic procedures [14–16]. Analysis of data from experiments has demonstrated the following:

- The safest slipknots are the Meltzer, Tayside, and Roeder knots by using use braided suture materials, such as Dacron (Ethibond, Ti-Cron, and Ethiflex) and Lactomer (Polysorb, Dexon, and Vicryl).
- The Aberdeen knot has been shown to be stronger and more secure than a surgeon's knot for ending a suture line [17].
- Compared to Roeder knot, Meltzer knot is more secure, but harder to tie than Roeder knot.
- The holding strengths of the cross, square, and blood knots are weak with all ligature materials tested, why we did not introduce them in paragraph "different knots."
- Polydioxanone is a safe ligature material for the Meltzer and Tayside but not the Roeder knot.
- Extracorporeal slipknots tied with silk and polyamides are less secure than the equivalent knots with Dacron, Lactomer, and polydioxanone.

The results of in vitro studies suggested that the Roeder and fisherman's knots were the least secure of all laparoscopic knots in all sutures tested, with the exception

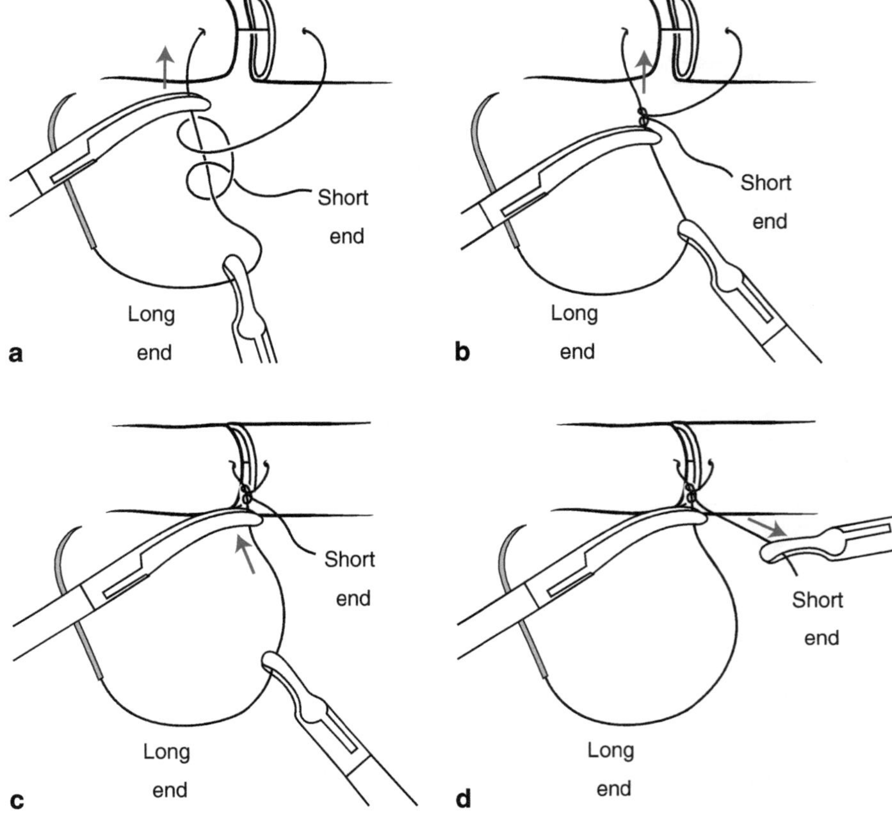

Fig. 9.14 (**a–d**) Make a square knot as slipknot

of polyglactin tied with a fisherman's knot, which was as secure as the extracorporeal and intracorporeal polyglactin knots. These experiments showed laparoscopic square knots to be as secure as open square knots; removing the operating finger from the knot does not seem to affect the security of a well-tied square knot. Furthermore, of the permanent sutures tested, there was no substantive difference in the security of laparoscopic intracorporeally and extracorporeally tied knots. Silk is, however, not as secure as other permanent suture materials. Amortegui et al. [18] compared seven types of knots, and the conclusion was: all knots must be made with six throws because security is maximized (Fig. 9.15).

9.5 Different Sutures

9.5.1 Instruments

Nowadays, there are a variety of suturing devices and self-righting needle drivers are available. Here, I would like to introduce some of them. One general principle is

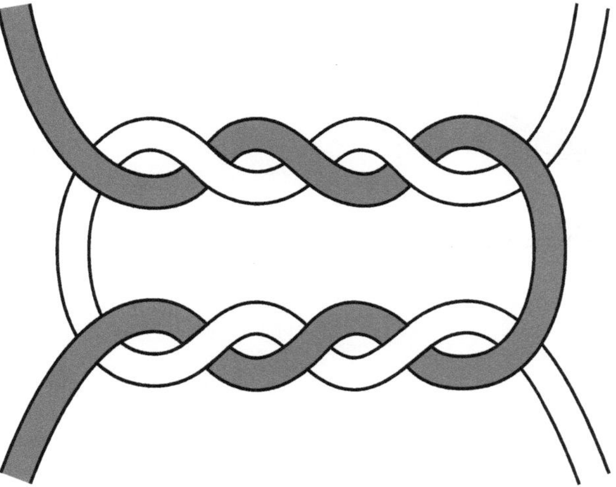

Fig. 9.15 Six throws are needed to make a maximal security

that two needle drives are needed because two-handed laparoscopic suturing is an essential skill for the advanced laparoscopist.

9.5.1.1 Needle Holder (Fig. 9.16)

The perfect needle holder should be ergonomic, light, and have a hard needle grip and at the same time easy to change needle positioning. However, such kind of needle holder is not easy to find.

They were in part insufficient in terms of weight, handgrips, tips, and movement possibilities. Newly developed suture devices, disposable and reusable, made intracorporeal suturing easier, but they are still not satisfactory in terms of size, needle design, and economic properties [19–22]. Therefore, the main attention of new suture devices should be directed toward these problems.

9.5.1.2 Endo Stitch Laparoscopic Suturing Device (Fig. 9.17)

This suturing device can combine with a running or interrupted stitches in soft tissues and locked suture technique with Lap Tie or Hem-o-lok to achieve a rapid hemostatic, clinically secure closure especially in pyeloplasty surgery and partial nephrectomy. The advantage of this device is it is a proprietary toggle-activated, needle-passing technology that eliminates the need to load and unload the needle while passing it through tissue. This feature can potentially provide significant OR time savings during laparoscopic procedures when compared with needle drivers. It can be used with one hand with advantage in single port laparoscopic surgery. The step-by-step Endo Stitch is shown in Fig. 9.18a, b.

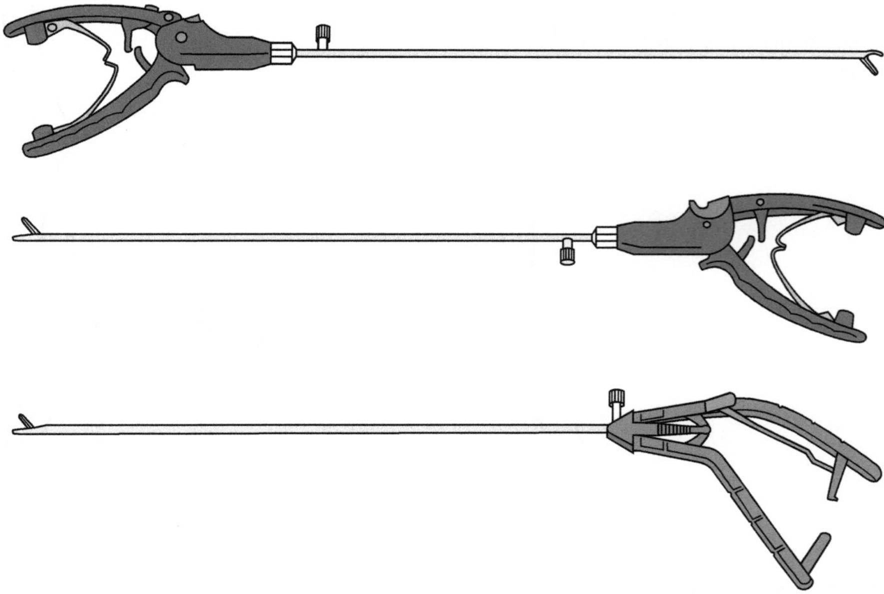

Fig. 9.16 Different needle holders

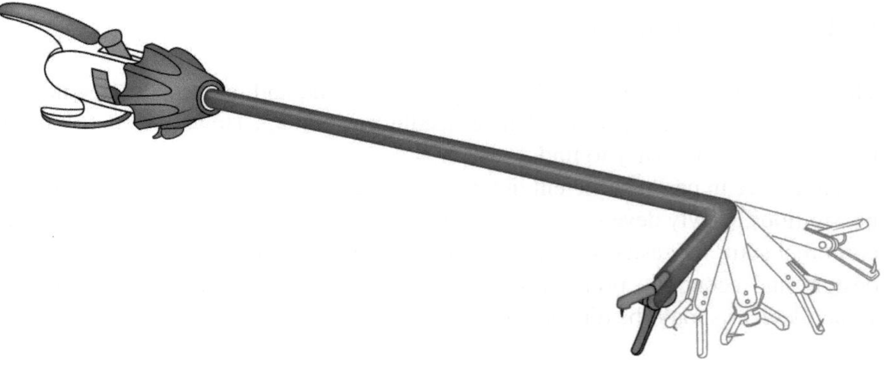

Fig. 9.17 Endo Stitch laparoscopic suturing device

9.5.2 *Sling Suture (Fig. 9.19a–d)*

This technique has been described by Nathanson and Cuschieri. In the multiple puncture technique for intra-abdominal surgery, active bleeding from the abdominal wall may be encountered. This bleeding can be controlled by a sling suture. This way may be effective in this situation [23].

9.5.3 Continuous Suture (Fig. 9.20a–c)

There are some different means about continuous suturing.

The technique of suturing is like the usual continuous suture except for the use of metal clip as a knot at the beginning and the end of suture. This way is usually used in partial nephrectomy [11].

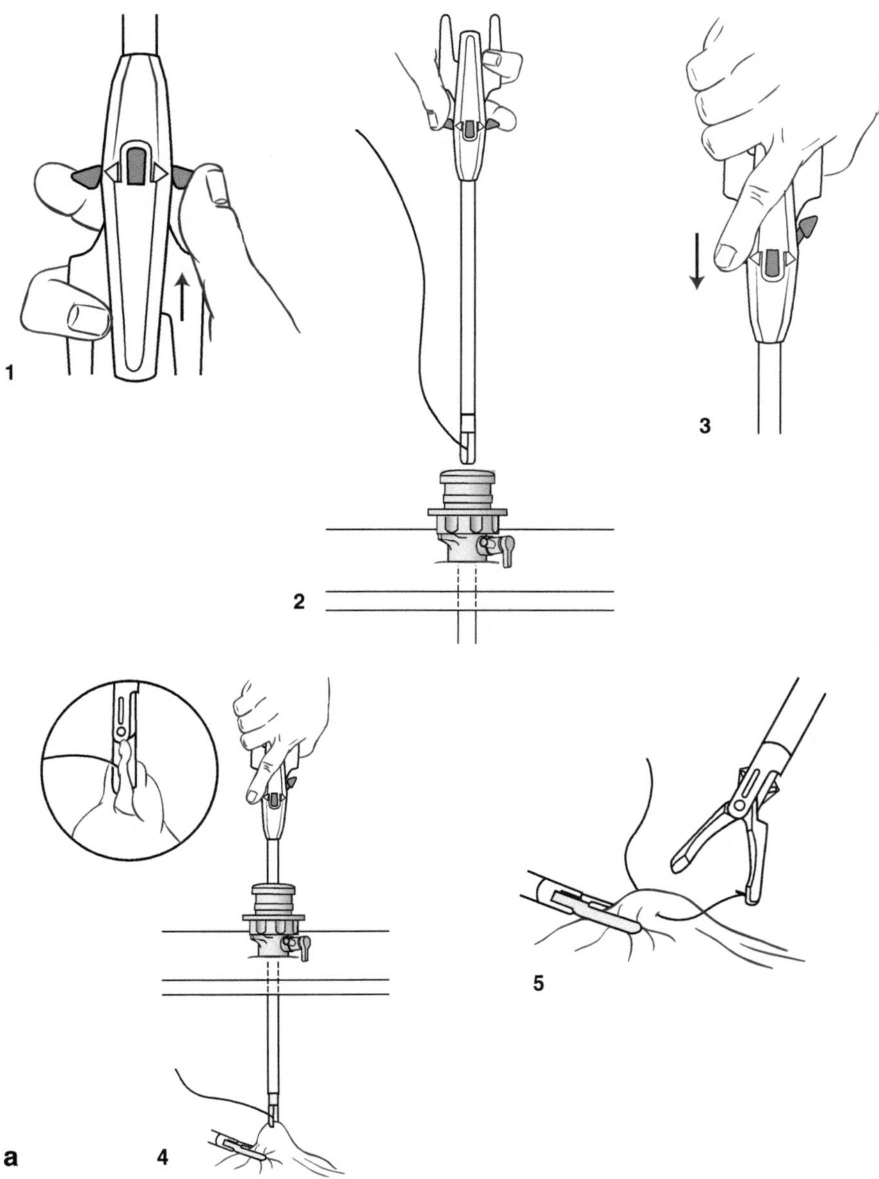

Fig. 9.18 (**a**) Introducing of Endo Stitch laparoscopic suturing device. (**b**) Using Endo Stitch laparoscopic suturing device intracorporeally

Fig. 9.18 (continued)

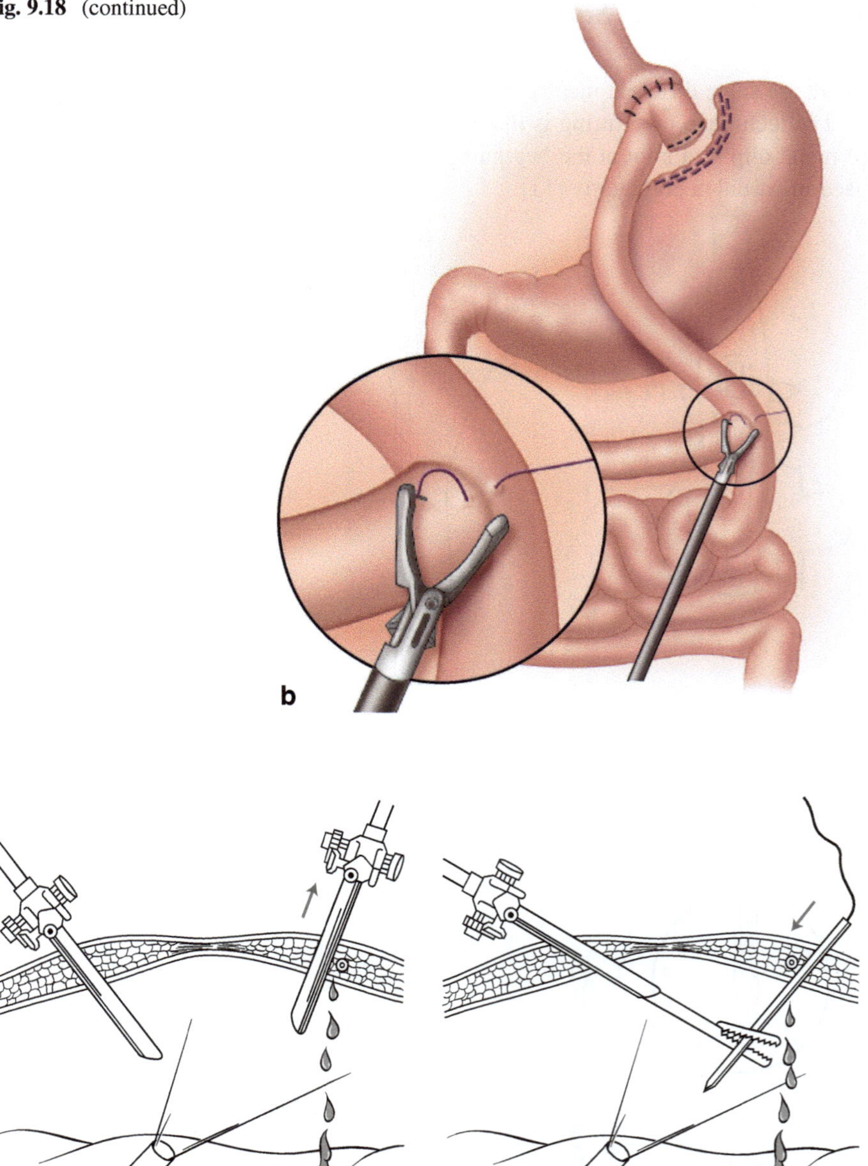

Fig. 9.19 (**a**–**d**) Sling suture in practicing

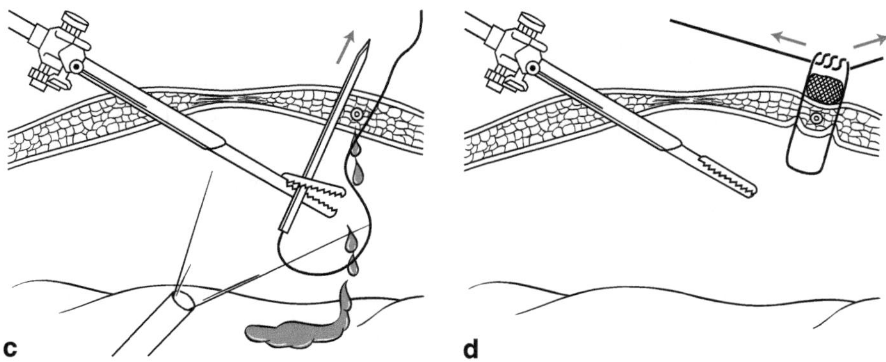

Fig. 9.19 (continued)

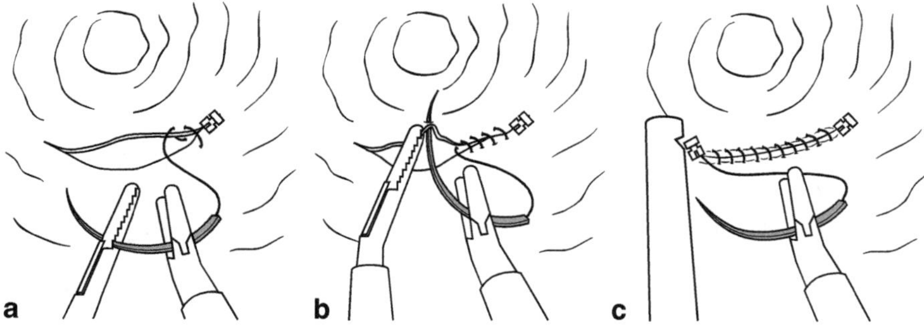

Fig. 9.20 (**a**–**c**) Continuous suture

A special way to do continuous suture is introduced to make vesicourethral anastomosis in radical prostatectomy by Van Velthoven 2003 [24] (Fig. 9.21a–d).

9.6 Laparoscopic Suture Techniques

9.6.1 Needle Positioning

It can be a difficult, frustrating, and time-consuming step with needle positioning during laparoscopic suturing. The problems of intracorporeal suturing are mainly caused by nonsuturing activities (i.e., handling of the curved needle, stitching accurately). Following, we would like to show some tricks concerning needle positioning. The ground principle is that optimal angle between the tip of the needle holder and the needle should be around 90° (Fig. 9.22).

Furthermore, Brody et al. presented a reliable and efficient technique for laparoscopic needle positioning (Fig. 9.23):

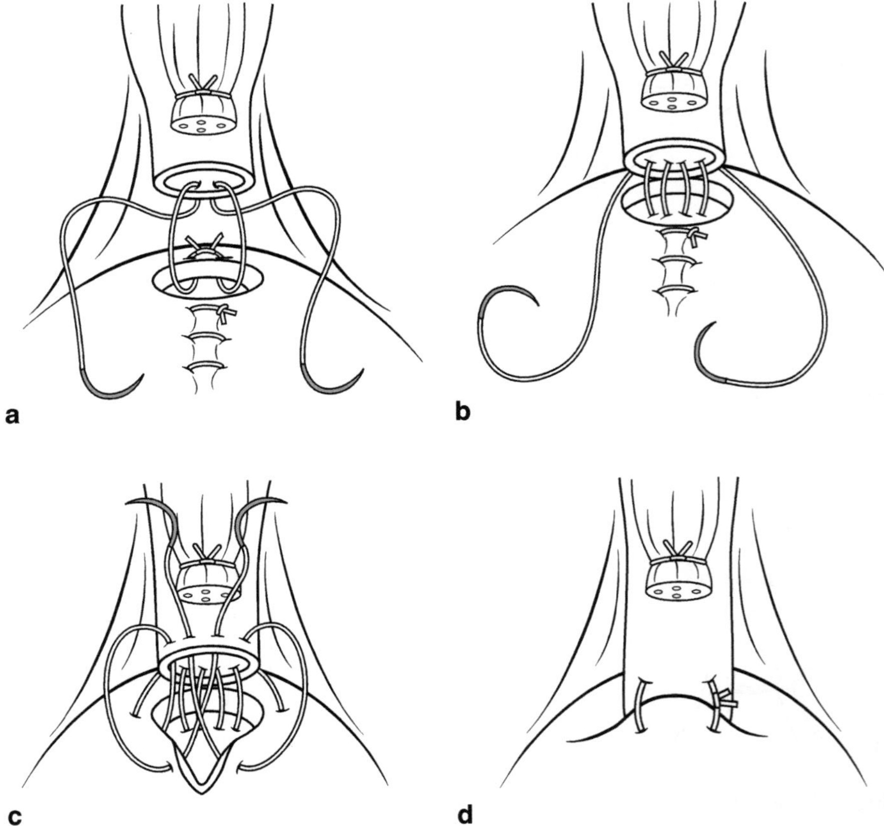

Fig. 9.21 Van Velthoven technique for performing the running single knot anastomosis. (**a**) The two sutures, which were knotted together extracorporeally, have been passed outside-in on the bladder and inside-out on the urethra at the 5:30 and 6:30 o'clock positions, respectively. (**b**) One suture is run clockwise and the opposite suture is run counterclockwise to the 9:00 and 3:00 o'clock positions to make background of anastomosis water tight. (**c**) Similar transition stitch will be continually done in the foreground. (**d**) As a result of the transition stitches, the single intracorporeal knot resides on the outside of the bladder

- For right-handed insertion, the needle is back loaded and introduced through the trocar.
- The needle holder rotates in a clockwise direction so the needle concavity points toward 6 o'clock.
- The left-handed needle holder grasps the needle at its midpoint and rotates counterclockwise. The needle concavity now points toward 12 o'clock.
- The needle is grasped and ready for suturing.
- For a left-handed insertion, the needle is back loaded as before and inserted. The left-handed needle holder rotates in a clockwise direction.

The needle concavity is now pointing toward 12 o'clock and simply grasped at the appropriate position.

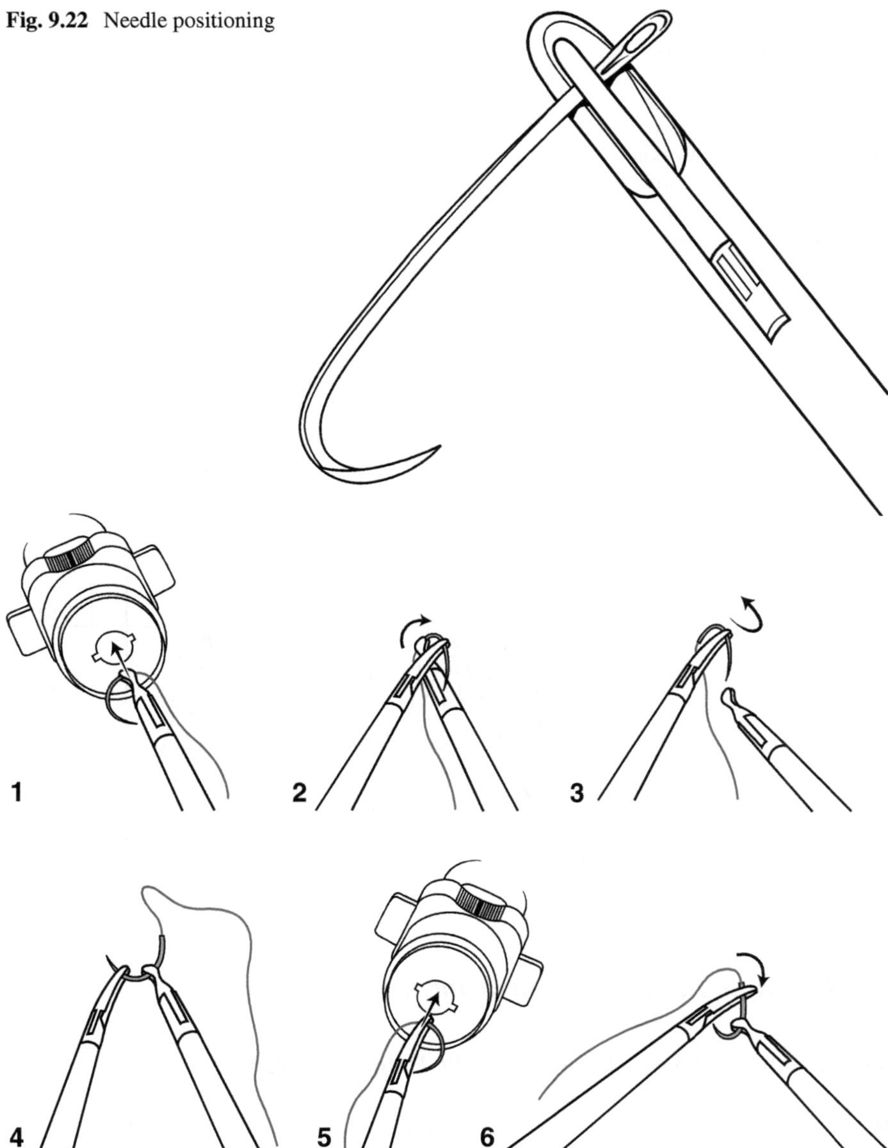

Fig. 9.22 Needle positioning

Fig. 9.23 Changing needle positions intracorporeally

9.6.2 Space Between Trocars

To avoid an acute angle between the instruments, a distance between the trocars should be 15–20 cm [25], which is hard to realize during retroperitoneoscopy. For anastomosis suturing, optimal distance between trocars is 12 cm.

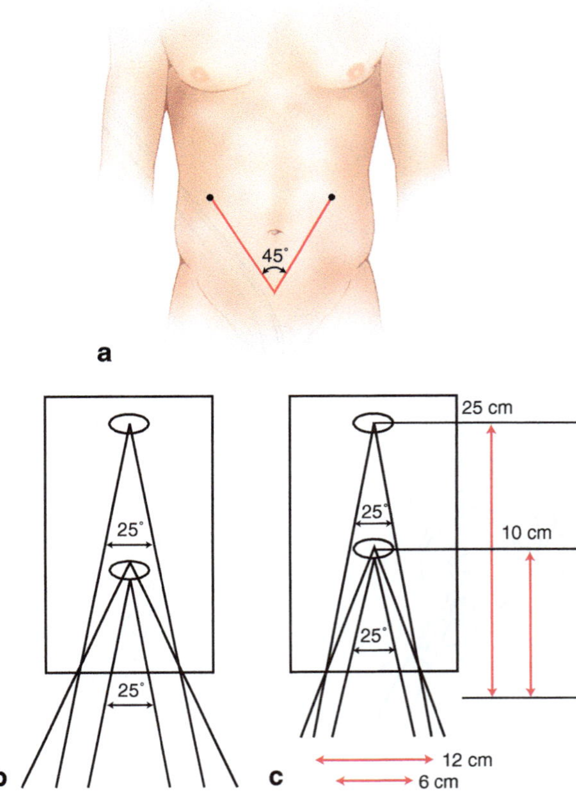

Fig. 9.24 (**a**) Optimal angle between needle holders is <45°. (**b, c**) A long intracorporeal length of the instruments allows a great distance between the working ports; consequently, a short intracorporeal instrument length requires a reduction of the distance between the working ports

9.6.3 *Angle Between the Instruments*

9.6.3.1 Optimal Angle Between Needle Holders Is <45°

We recommend an angle of <45 ° between the instruments. These differences in recommendations can be explained, apart from different suturing techniques, by the special requirements of reconstructive endoscopy in retroperitoneoscopy compared with transperitoneal laparoscopy. Results revealed, as Frede and Rassweiler [10], an angle of <45 ° is necessary to maintain optimal access for intracorporeal suturing. A short intracorporeal length of the instruments, together with a greater distance between the working ports, means an obtuse angle between the instruments, which makes reconstructive surgery technically more difficult. Therefore, the distance between the working ports should be chosen according to the intracorporeal length of the instruments to create an angle of <45 ° between the instruments. A long intracorporeal length of the instruments allows a great distance between the working ports; consequently, a short intracorporeal instrument length requires a reduction of the distance between the working ports (Fig. 9.24a–c).

Meanwhile,suturing objects in the lateral position always means a more acute angle and a lesser distance between the instruments compared with suturing objects in a central position.

9.6.3.2 Angle Between the Instruments and the Horizontal Line

The results of an in vivo experiment has been shown, as noted by Pier and associates, that suturing in more horizontal positions between the instruments and a horizontal line is easier than suturing in more vertical positions. The reasons for this are the difficulties in the handling of the instruments in vertical positions and the force of gravity. Therefore, the operation table position should be changed during surgery according to the requirements. Optimal angle between needle holders and anastomosis is 55° (Fig. 9.25a–c).

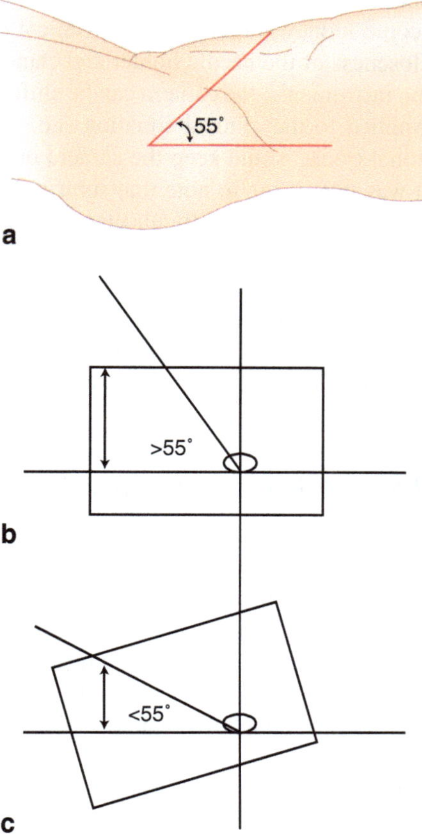

Fig. 9.25 **(a–c)** Optimal angle between needle holders and anastomosis is 55°

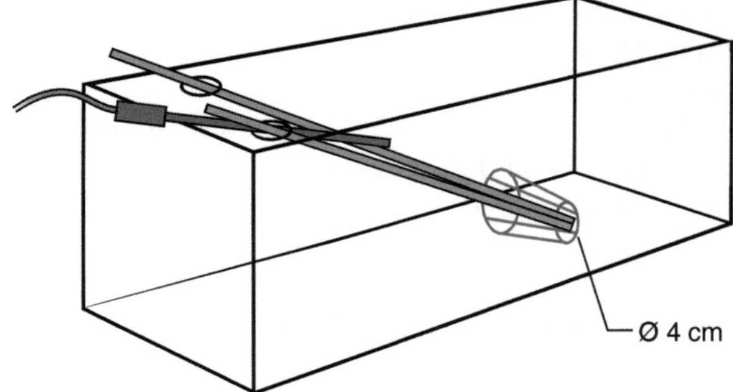

Fig. 9.26 Training suturing in a box with maximally narrowed space

9.6.4 *Flexible Camera Position*

The relation between the instruments and the camera will be kept constant, as will the angle between the instruments; thus, the movement of the instruments will not be hindered by the camera. This skill enhances fluency between clutching, optimizing hand position, camera movement, and suturing. In cases of limited space between the working trocars and lateral positions of the object (i.e., retroperitoneoscopic kidney surgery), the movement of the instruments can be hindered by the closeness of the needle holder and camera. To get more space for the movement of the instruments, the camera can be shifted into a position contralateral to the object. Applied to the clinical situation (i.e., retroperitoneoscopic pyeloplasty), an additional trocar would keep the camera out of the working field (site of anastomosis). It was interesting to note that suturing in a position left lateral to the working port seemed to be more difficult than suturing in right lateral positions. One reason for this is the proximity of the needle holder and the camera for right-handed surgeons when working in a left lateral position. The movement of the needle holder is often restricted by the camera. Consequently, suturing in the right lateral positions of the camera is much easier for right-handed surgeons. So it is very important to keep flexible camera position in laparoscopy.

9.6.5 *When in a Maximally Narrowed Space (Fig. 9.26)*

Even suturing in a maximally narrowed space (max. diameter of 4 cm vs. 25 cm available for the movement of the instruments) was possible, provided there was a standardized suturing technique, training, and optimal geometric conditions. To avoid problems handling the suture filament in these limited conditions, the filament length should not exceed 10 cm (thread length may be 10–15 cm generally), which is still long enough to create one complete single knot.

Acknowledgements Dr Zhu Qinyi, Dept of Urology, Jiansu TMC Hospital, Nanjing, China.

References

1. Clayman RV, Kavoussi LR, Soper NJ, et al. Laparoscopic nephrectomy: initial case report. J Urol. 1991;146:278–82.
2. Bowersox JC, Cornum RL. Remote operative urology using a surgical telemanipulator system: preliminary observations. Urology. 1998;52:17–22.
3. Ahlering TE, Skarecky D, Lee D, et al. Successful transfer of open surgical skills to a laparoscopic environment using a robotic interface: initial experience with laparoscopic radical prostatectomy. J Urol. 2003;170:1738–41.
4. Peña González JA, Pascual Queralt M, Salvador Bayarri JT, et al. Evolution of open versus laparoscopic/robotic surgery: 10 years of changes in urology. Actas Urol Esp. 2010;34:223–31.
5. Ronney A. The robotic surgery era and the role of laparoscopy training. Ther Adv Urol. 2009;1:161–5.
6. Gomez MS, Baig MM, Muskovich JA, et al. Contribution of laparoscopic training to robotic proficiency. JSLS. 2008;12:S66.
7. Resad P, Ronald L. Laparoscopic suturing and ligation techniques. J Am Assoc Gynecol Laparosc. 1995;3:67–79.
8. Croce E, Olmi S. Intracorporeal knot-tying and suturing techniques in laparoscopic surgery: technical details. JSLS. 2000;4:17–22.
9. Klaiber C, Metzger A. Manual der laparoskopischen chirurgie. Bern: Huber, Ko ST, Airan MC.Therapeutic laparoscopic suturing techniques. Surg Endosc. 1992;6:41–6.
10. Frede T, Stock C, Renner C, et al. Geometry of laparoscopic suturing and knotting techniques. J Endourol. 1999;13:191–9.
11. Sung Ko ST, Airan MC. Therapeutic laparoscopic suturing techniques. Surg Endosc. 1992;6:41–6.
12. Barabás L, Sipos P. Laparoscopic knot tying. Magy. 2008;61:116–20.
13. Meng MV, Stoller ML. Laparoscopic intracorporeal square-to-slip knot. Urology. 2002;59:932–3.
14. Shimi SM, Lirici M, Vander Velpen G, et al. Comparative study of the holding strength of slipknots using absorbable and nonabsorbable ligature materials. Surg Endosc. 1994;8:1285–91.
15. Sedlack JD, Williams VM, DeSimone J, et al. Laparoscopic knot security. Surg Laparosc Endosc. 1996;6:144–6.
16. Rosin E, Robinson GM. Knot security of suture materials. Vet Surg. 1989;18:269–73.
17. Shaw AD, Duthie GS. A simple assessment of surgical sutures and knots. J R Coll Surg Edinb. 1995;40:388–91.
18. Amortegui JD, Restrepo H. Knot security in laparoscopic surgery – a comparative study with conventional knots. Surg Endosc. 2002;16:1598–602.
19. See WA, Cooper CS, Fisher RJ. Predictors of laparoscopic complications after formal training in laparoscopic surgery. JAMA. 1993;270:2689–92.
20. Kadirkamanthan SS, Shelton JC, Hepworth CC. A comparison of the strength of knots tied by hand and at laparoscopy. J Am Coll Surg. 1996;182:46–54.
21. Hamad MA, Mentges B, Schurr MO, et al. Laparoscopic intracorporeal bowel anastomosis by a new suturing device: a study in a laparoscopic simulator with integrated animal organs. Minim Invas Ther. 1997;6:296–303.
22. Frede T, Hatzinger M, Grenacher L. Experimental aspects of laparoscopic suturing and knotting techniques during retroperitoneoscopy (abstract). J Endourol. 1997;1 suppl 1:S54.
23. Nathanson LK, Cuschieri A. The falciform lift: a simple method for retraction of the falciform ligament during laparoscopic cholecystectomy. Surg Endosc. 1990;4:186.
24. Van Velthoven RF, Ahlering TE, Peltier A, et al. Technique for laparoscopic running urethrovesical anastomosis: the single knot method. Urology. 2003;61:699–702.
25. Pier A, Thevissen P, Eikel M. Laparoskopische Naht- und Knüpftechniken. Chirurg. 1994;65:473–83.

Chapter 10
Dissection and Hemostasis in Urologic Laparoscopy: Tips and Tricks

Jian Huang

Abstract The general principle of dissection in laparoscopic surgery is to be familiar with avascular anatomic planes of all kinds of urinary organs and every important anatomical landmark. Various options of hemostatic techniques (physical modalities, thermal modalities, and tissue sealants) can be employed in the laparoscopic approach, and timely surgical conversion should be always kept in mind. Local compression is the first step in the emergent management of bleeding and may be all that is needed in some cases. For larger vessels of up to 7 mm, LigaSure™ should be preferred, but below 4 mm, all vessel sealing systems seem to be equivalent. Any device with thermal diffusion should be completely avoided when nerve-sparing surgery is attempted.

Keywords Urology • Laparoscopy • Surgery • Technique • Tips • Tricks

10.1 Introduction

Dissection and hemostasis represent two important parts of any laparoscopic procedures.

In contrast to open surgery, laparoscopic dissection presents several limitations. High-quality video image is essential to deal with the two-dimensional space, and surgeons should take care about meticulous hemostasis as small bleedings can rapidly reduce the quality of the video image and ultimately impair surgical vision, with a potential direct impact on the safety and quality of the operation [1].

On the other hand, charring due to excessive coagulation will also decrease the vision through light absorption by dark areas and changes in the aspect of tissues.

J. Huang, M.D., Ph.D.
Department of Urology, Sun Yat-sen Memorial Hospital, Sun Yat-sen University, Yanjiang Xi Road, GhuangDong, GuangZhou 510120, China
e-mail: yehjn@yahoo.com.cn

Y.H. Sun et al. (eds.), *The Training Courses of Urological Laparoscopy*,
DOI 10.1007/978-1-4471-2723-9_10, © Springer-Verlag London 2012

10.2 General Principles of Dissection in Laparoscopic Surgery

The surgeon should be familiar with the vascular anatomic plane of all kinds of urinary organs and every important anatomical landmark. Putting the dissecting tissue on stretch and keeping proper tension can facilitate surgical procedures. Sharp dissection often is preferred by surgeons in most cases, as laparoscopy allows them to see very nicely where to cut [2].

Around great vessels and major organs, blunt dissection can be effectively performed by using the suction device [3]. As mentioned by Dr. Rassweiler, what one has to learn from the beginning is the "one hand feeds the other technique." Whatever you do, keep the image still. And then one hand feeds the other.

When encountering bothersome oozing or bleeding during dissection, packing gauze is particularly useful to absorb blood or other fluids. The gauze can be cut to the required length and easily inserted through one of the ports.

10.3 Dissection During Upper Urinary Tract Laparoscopic Surgery: Tips and Tricks

10.3.1 Transperitoneal Approach

During transperitoneal laparoscopic nephrectomy, it is very important for the novice laparoscopic surgeon to recognize the plane between the mesentery of the colon and anterior Gerota's fascia. By correctly identifying that plane, any violation to the mesentery is avoided.

After reflecting the bowel medially, the ureter and gonadal veins are identified and retracted laterally, and the psoas muscle is identified between the ipsilateral great vessel medially and the ureter/gonadal vein laterally.

On the left side, the gonadal vein is then traced cephalad to identify the renal vein. Following the gonadal vein cephalad is the best way to identify the left renal vein.

A clip is first placed on the renal artery to occlude the arterial flow to the kidney. Thereafter, the renal vein is taken with Hem-o-lok™. The renal artery is now clearly visualized and dissected, and additional clips are placed and transected [4].

On the right side, the gonadal vein enters the vena cava and can be clipped and divided to prevent inadvertent injury. Along the vena cava, the renal vein can be found and then is taken on the left side, and finally the renal artery is secured.

A very simple technique to find and dissect the ureter from the fat of the retroperitoneal space is to first identify and then lift the lower pole of the kidney, putting it on stretch and thereby exposing the space which is medial to it (Fig. 10.1). In doing so, you can lift the ureter and the hilum away from the colon and the great vessels so that further dissection is much easier.

Another simple technique is to leave the ureter intact during the dissection so that you do not have to spend a grasper or tractor on the cut end of the ureter during a nephrectomy. However, if the ureter is left intact, a blunt instrument can be simply

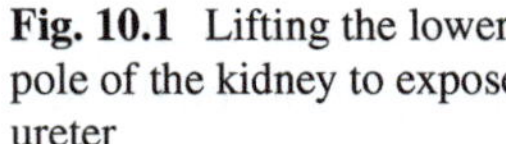
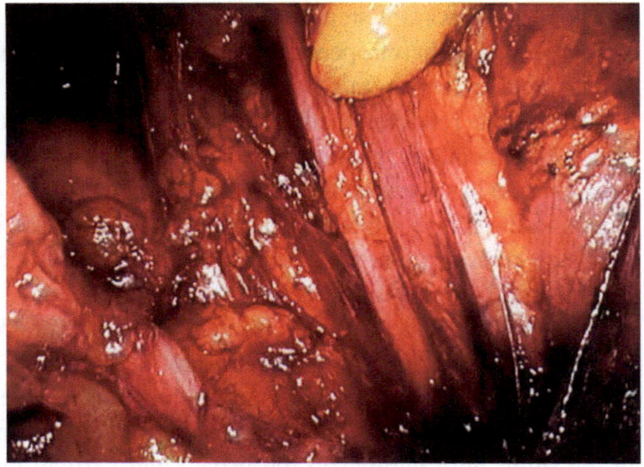

Fig. 10.1 Lifting the lower pole of the kidney to expose ureter

used to lift the ureter so that the hilum can be put on stretch. This also prevents loss of orientation and twisting of the kidney.

When performing transperitoneal laparoscopic adrenal surgery, how to expose the gland and central vein is the key point. On the left side, it is important to obtain wide exposure of the adrenal gland by adequately mobilizing the spleen. This is done by dividing the peritoneal attachments of the spleen all the way to the greater curvature of the stomach. Once adequately mobilized, the spleen falls away from the operative field and provides excellent exposure of the upper pole of the kidney and adrenal. The landmarks around the upper pole of the kidney including the diaphragm, transversus muscle, and quadratus lumborum muscle are identified, and medial to the adrenal, the posterior surface of the pancreas is identified. Following delineation of the above structures, the adrenal vein can be identified. However, if the adrenal vein is to be identified early, one can dissect close to the renal hilum, opening the Gerota's fascia. The renal vein can be then identified and then the adrenal vein along its upper border. But, unless indicated, the preference is to dissect and secure the adrenal vein last in order to prevent congestion of the adrenal gland.

On the right side, it is fairly easy to identify the adrenal vein. The peritoneum between the liver and the kidney is divided and then an additional incision alongside the inferior vena cava is made. The upper half of the kidney is exposed. The liver is retracted with a retractor. The renal vein is easily identified draining into the vena cava. Then, dissecting along the vena cava toward the liver, the right adrenal gland can be found. The vena cava is an important landmark. The short hepatic vein that drains into the vena cava is a good guide to the adrenal vein as it lies very close to it and is almost at the same level.

10.3.2 Retroperitoneal Approach

The retroperitoneal approach provides a more direct access for renal and adrenal gland laparoscopic surgery.

The most important step during laparoscopic kidney surgery is how to find and handle the hilum. In retroperitoneoscopic renal surgery, after port placement, the first step is to place the Gerota's fascia-covered kidney on significant lateral traction with a laparoscopic retractor in the surgeon's nondominant hand. Using a suction or J-hook electrocautery, gentle dissection is performed along the anterior surface of the psoas muscle in superomedial direction. At this point, it is important to keep the dissection in the flimsy white fibroareolar tissue along the ipsilateral great vessel. One must stay anterior to the ipsilateral great vessel, taking care not to stray posteriorly. Again, good lateral countertraction is important to place the renal hilum on stretch.

In general, the renal hilum is located at an angle of 45–60 degrees from the vertical axis. The renal artery is posterior, and the renal vein is anterior and usually caudal (inferior) to the renal artery. Before beginning dissection on the renal artery or vein, the horizontal positions of the major vessels (aorta on the left side, vena cava on the right: both parallel to the psoas) and vertical pulsations of the fat-covered renal artery laterally are looked for and almost always visualized.

One must remember that, during renal retroperitoneoscopy, the psoas is the constant anatomic landmark: the psoas "is your best friend."

For adrenal surgery, especially for adrenal masses with a significant retrocaval component, the retroperitoneal approach can be regarded as a better option. Dissection along fat planes surrounding the adrenal mass is safe. Bleeding from adrenal parenchyma laceration would disturb the procedure. During laparoscopic adrenalectomy, there is usually no need to identify the adrenal artery. Adrenal arteries are usually arborizations of vessels coming from a variety of areas. The vast majority can be dissected with a hook cautery or the harmonic scalpel. There is a 10% incidence of an aberrant adrenal vein coming directly from the liver into the adrenal on the right side. Because of this, one needs to be more cautious on the right side. It is important to secure the aberrant adrenal vein by using the harmonic scalpel or clip ligation. Additionally, for large adrenal masses extending posterior to the renal hilum, one needs to be careful not to accidentally misrecognize and transect a segmental renal artery for the adrenal artery (Fig. 10.2).

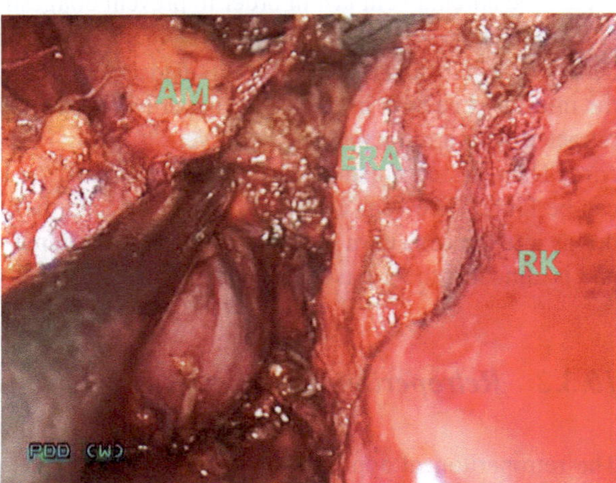

Fig. 10.2 Ectopic renal segmental artery during right laparoscopic adrenalectomy. *AM* adrenal mass, *ERA* ectopic renal artery, *RK* right kidney

10.4 Dissection During Lower Urinary Tract Laparoscopic Surgery: Tips and Tricks

In case of laparoscopic procedures on lower urinary tract organs, including bladder and prostate, exposure and dissection of tissues become very difficult because of limited space and disturbance of intestine. A steep Trendelenburg position is essential to keep the bowel out of the pelvis during surgery.

Laparoscopic radical cystectomy usually starts by visualizing the pelvis and releasing adhesions of the sigmoid colon to the pelvic side wall. This mobilization of the sigmoid allows retraction out of the pelvis and identification of the left ureter and assists in the subsequent lymphadenectomy. If the sigmoid continues to fall into the pelvis, it can be held in place by a suture placed through an appendix epiploica and held to the abdominal wall.

At this time, the major landmarks in the pelvis should be visualized. These are the ureters, medial umbilical ligaments, vasa deferentia, and urachus. The tip of the urethral catheter is also frequently seen in the bladder dome.

The ureters can be first dissected and mobilized distally toward the bladder. Proximal dissection to a level above the iliac vessels greatly facilitates the subsequent lymphadenectomy and the urinary diversion. The ureters are then divided distally close to the bladder with LigaSure™ instead of clips [5, 6].

Pelvic lymphadenectomy involving large lymphatic vessels using LigaSure™ can reduce lymphatic fluid spillage and therefore minimize the risk of lymphocele.

Important dissection planes during radical cystectomy are the posterior plane between the seminal vesicles and prostate anteriorly and the rectal wall posteriorly, as well as the lateral plane, between the bladder within the perivesical fat and the pelvic side wall including the iliac vessels, obturator fossa, and pelvic floor muscles. These planes are generally avascular. Thus, understanding and meticulously following them are essential for a technically and oncologically sound operation.

The posterior plane usually is developed first, keeping the bladder attached to the anterior abdominal wall to allow exposure. Following the vas deferens medially can facilitate identifying this plane in difficult cases. The tips of the seminal vesicles are visualized easily, and keeping the seminal vesicles anterior, the plane is developed distally toward the prostate. Denonvilliers' fascia is encountered at the level of the prostatovesical junction posteriorly. This fascia needs to be divided sharply, allowing the posterior plane to be developed further distally between the prostate and the anterior rectal surface. Extreme care should be exercised at this time to avoid injuring the rectum.

The lateral planes then are developed distally into the pelvis until the pelvic floor muscle and the endopelvic fascia are reached. The reflection of the endopelvic fascia over the prostate can be divided. The posterolateral bladder pedicles thus are exposed between the posterior and lateral planes. These pedicles usually are divided with LigaSure™.

After mobilizing the bladder from the anterior abdominal wall, the space of Retzius is developed, and the puboprostatic ligaments are exposed. The superficial branch of the dorsal vein is coagulated and divided with LigaSure™. The dorsal vein can be controlled by a controlling stitch. A locking clip or a suture should be placed at the proximal urethra to prevent tumor spillage from the bladder when the urethra is divided. Proximal traction on the prostatic apex through inflated Foley catheter facilitates the dissection of posterior wall of urethra.

For nerve-sparing cystoprostatectomy, both ureters are dissected, clipped, and transected at the bladder. A posterior horizontal peritoneotomy is made in the rectovesical cul-de-sac. The Denonvilliers' fascia is opened, and a plane is created between the bladder and rectum. Dissection is performed in the midline, immediately along the posterior surface of the seminal vesicles and vasa deferentia, which were maintained en bloc with the specimen. Electrocautery or ultrasound energy is not used at any point in the vicinity of the neurovascular bundles (NVBs), which run along the tip and lateral surface of the seminal vesicle up to the prostatovesical junction. In the nerve-sparing technique, the dissection proceeds closer to the bladder and further from the rectum. The NVBs are sequentially teased away with cold cutting, and hemostasis is secured with Hem-o-lok™ clips. The posterior peritoneotomy is then extended anteriorly, and the prevesical space of Retzius is developed.

The endopelvic fascia is maintained intact bilaterally, and the lateral pelvic fascia is incised high along the prostate to release and drop the NVBs posteriorly. The dorsal vein complex can be secured with a stitch, exposing the urethra. The NVBs are released from the prostatic apex using cold incision, and the urethra is divided after both NVBs are completely mobilized.

Likewise, during laparoscopic radical prostatectomy, in terms of dissecting and preserving the neurovascular bundles, antegrade dissection of the neurovascular bundles may be preferred because it follows in line with the path of the nerve bundles from the seminal vesicle to the prostatic apex. The antegrade technique also allows for early ligation of the prostatic pedicles and late division of the dorsal venous complex, which are two major sources of bleeding. This results in minimal blood loss during the more difficult steps of neurovascular bundle preservation.

The key point is to identify the proper plane of dissection between the lateral pelvic fascia and the prostatic fascia. The NVBs lie between these two periprostatic tissue planes. Thus, by incising the outer lateral pelvic fascia, the surgeon is allowed to identify the NVBs and tease the nerve fibers away from the inner prostatic fascia. With this step, a lateral NVB groove is developed. It can serve as an excellent landmark guiding the surgeon during antegrade dissection and preservation of the NVBs from the base to the apex of the prostate. The apical dissection of the NVB is typically the most challenging step as the nerve closely approximates the prostatic apex at the prostatourethral junction. By leaving this step at the end, after complete dissection of the prostate, the prostate is now more mobile, which helps to improve visualization of the precise course of NVBs and facilitates their release and preservation at the apex.

10.5 Hemostasis in Urologic Laparoscopy: Tips and Tricks

Adequate hemostasis is essential during advanced laparoscopic procedures since uncontrolled bleeding may cause significant complications and even require conversion to laparotomy to obtain sufficient hemostasis.

Although as troublesome as with open surgery, the problem of intraoperative bleeding is compounded by aspects that are proper to laparoscopic surgery, such as the inability to have direct manual access to the bleeding site for compression and the loss of visibility due to light absorption by the surrounding blood.

In addition, laparoscopic intracorporeal knot tying can be a complex task in certain situations, especially in the presence of active bleeding, and this is especially true for the novice surgeon [7].

Nonetheless, many of the hemostatic techniques used in the laparoscopic approach were adapted from open surgery, and the basic surgical principles of prevention and proper surgical technique remain valid with both approaches.

10.5.1 General Management of Hemorrhage

Once bleeding has been temporarily reduced using compression, one of many available options can be used for definitive hemostatic control. These options include physical modalities, thermal modalities, and tissue sealants.

10.5.1.1 Physical Modalities

Standard surgical principles, such as proper tissue dissection and identification of supplying blood vessels, are used also in laparoscopy, allowing early identification of anatomical structures and timely implementation of appropriate measures, preferably before bleeding occurs.

Dissection either with a sponge or a hemostyptic stick helps to dissect tissue and to control blood vessels locally. Local compression with a sponge is similar to digital compression in open surgery, particularly with uncontrollable venous bleeding, and gives the surgeon time to elaborate further strategies for final hemostasis. Otherwise, local compression alone may be sufficient for hemostasis (Fig. 10.3).

Control of Santorini plexus during laparoscopic radical prostatectomy or cystectomy may pose a significant problem when massive hemorrhage occurs. Simple local compression by balloon catheter retraction for temporary occlusion has proven to be an excellent emergency measure (Fig. 10.4).

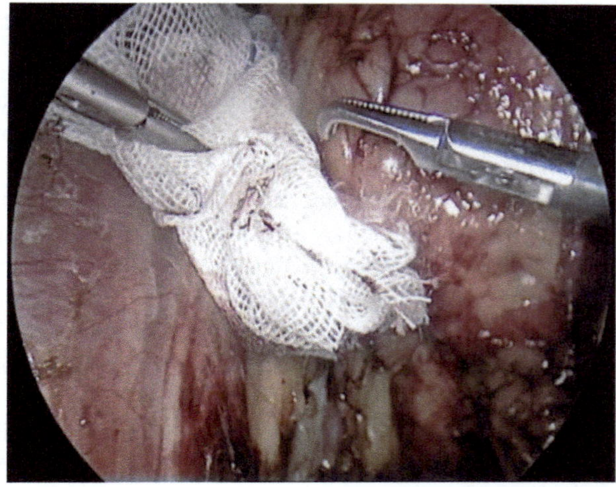

Fig. 10.3 Hemostasis by compressing with a laparoscopic sponge stick

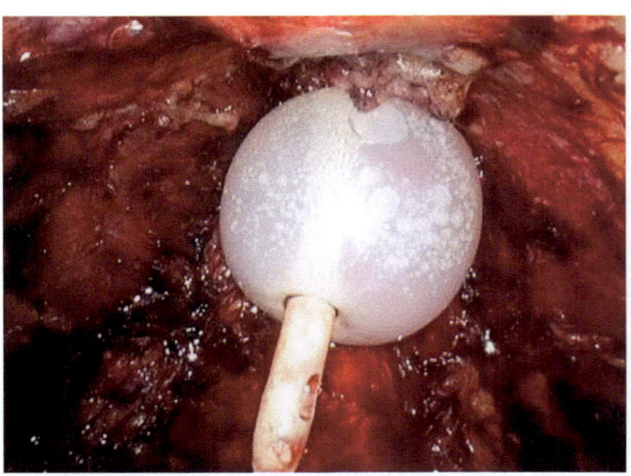

Fig. 10.4 Compression of Santorini plexus by catheter balloon retraction

Sutures remain a very effective hemostatic tool in laparoscopic surgery, just as with open surgery. Situations where freehand suture ligation may be used in laparoscopy include control of Santorini plexus during radical prostatectomy (Fig. 10.5) and parenchymal repair in partial nephrectomy (Fig. 10.6).

Since suturing requires advanced laparoscopic skills, clip systems represent a preferable method of sealing blood vessels. A wide variety of 5- and 10-mm clip appliers with various sized clips are available. Even reusable clip appliers and flexible instruments are available. However, the reloading time of such instruments can represent an important limitation in emergency situations.

In addition, titanium clips tend to slip off during further dissection. Consequently, at least 2–5 clips seem mandatory for safe control of >3-mm vessels. The self-locking, polymer ligation clip system (Hem-o-lok™) contains a self-sealing mechanism when correctly applied (Fig. 10.7). Therefore, these clips seem to have fewer

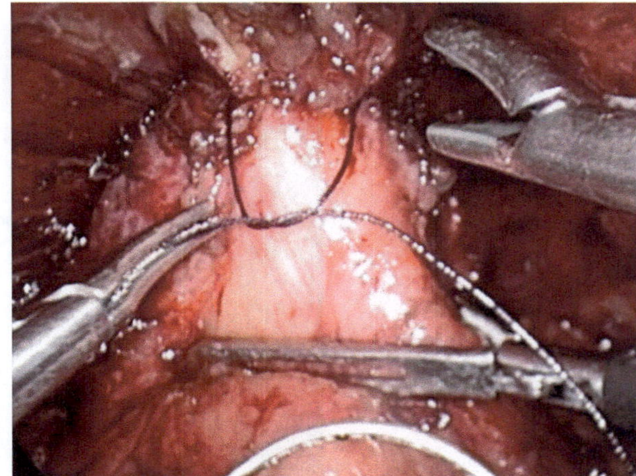

Fig. 10.5 Suture ligation of the Santorini plexus during laparoscopic radical prostatectomy or cystectomy

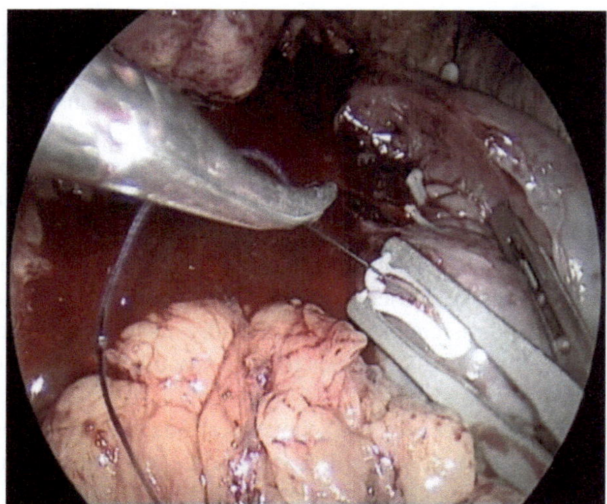

Fig. 10.6 Hemostasis achieved by intracorporeal suturing for renal parenchymal sealing

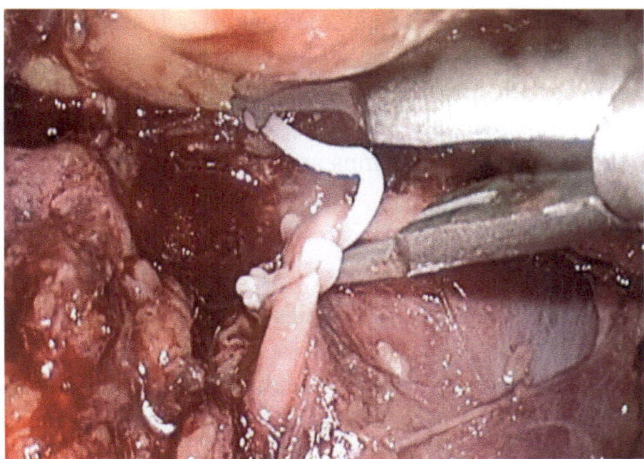

Fig. 10.7 The self-locking, polymer ligation clip system (Hem-o-lock)

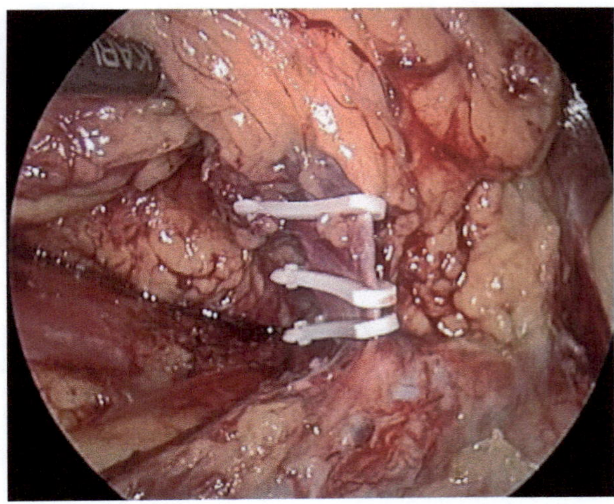

Fig. 10.8 Vascular control of renal pedicle by application of polymer ligation clips with the hook-like locking system (Hem-o-lock)

tendencies to slip off, compared with titanium clips, and therefore may be regarded as safer. Even major vessels, such as the renal vein or artery, can be safely controlled (Fig. 10.8).

In addition, locking clips are also used as suture bolsters in procedures such as partial nephrectomy, significantly reducing the time for parenchymal repair (Fig. 10.6).

Vascular endostapler (Endo-GIA) with 2.0- to 2.5-mm jaw width and various lengths has been used to achieve safe occlusion of major vessels or vascular pedicles. Modern endostaplers are bulky instruments, require 12-mm access ports, utilize three lines of staples for safe vascular control, and provide the cutting simultaneously [8, 9].

These devices require some educational training before use since the main reason for a "malfunction" is still inappropriate use of the instrument. The major disadvantage of endostaplers may occur when major vessels are sealed insufficiently, resulting in life-threatening bleeding. Consequently, the laparoscopic surgeon must first use the appropriate vascular jaw width (2.0–2.5 mm) and check that the entire vessel is within the stapler line before firing.

In certain situations where temporary control of large vessels is required, such as during laparoscopic partial nephrectomy, vascular clamps afford excellent control [10]. Laparoscopic clamps are available in the form of bulldog or Satinsky clamps (Fig. 10.9).

10.5.1.2 Thermal Modalities

Just as with the physical modalities, thermal modalities have been adapted from open surgery to serve the same purposes in laparoscopic surgery [11–13].

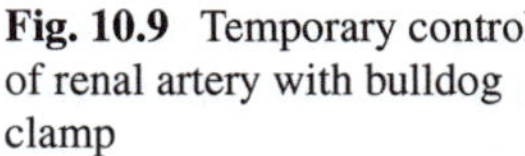

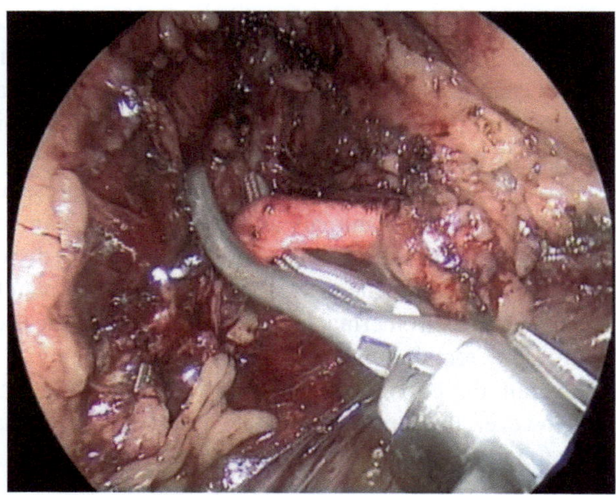

Fig. 10.9 Temporary control of renal artery with bulldog clamp

Predominant instruments used for monopolar dissection or cutting are forceps, scissors, or J-hook electrocautery. Monopolar instruments may be adequate for preventing or controlling minor superficial bleeding. In some cases, especially for avascular plane or tissue without key organs, dissection with J-hook using monopolar coagulation current may be an effective method for fast and efficient dissection and hemostasis. Monopolar instruments, however, have various disadvantages. One of them is the inappropriate current conduction which may lead to heat scatter with damage to adjacent organs.

Introduction of bipolar instruments, such as LigaSure™ and PlasmaKinetic™, in laparoscopy has improved safe dissection and hemostasis simultaneously, thus allowing early vascular and bleeding control while avoiding complications. The tools provide selective action on tissue contained between the forceps of the instrument, and scatter remains limited to a few millimeters, thus minimizing the risk of adjacent organ injury.

LigaSure™ has become a very popular instrument among laparoscopic surgeons. This instrument is FDA-approved for use on vessels less than 7 mm in diameter. It produces a hemostatic seal by applying energy that denatures the collagen and elastin in the vessel wall, and the pressure applied by the instrument imposes the walls, allowing the formation of a permanent seal. Comparative studies have shown that this seal may even be as effective as titanium clips for vessels in the range of 4–5 mm. It can also withstand supraphysiologic pressures (up to 442 mmHg) in the 6–7-mm vessel range.

The harmonic scalpel is a tool that simultaneously excises and coagulates tissue with high-frequency ultrasound. A frequency of 25 kHz results in dissection and cavitation. At >55 kHz, thermal effects and coagulation take place. The harmonic scalpel is known to cause less collateral damage, avoids carbonization of the tissue, and reduces local thermal damage. It has been used widely in laparoscopy for tissue dissection and control of local blood vessels. However, the use of harmonic scalpel is limited to vessels <4 mm, and complete hemostasis of larger vessels cannot be achieved. Since the immediate vascular control of all supplying vessels during dissection cannot be achieved, the use of the harmonic scalpel alone is not advisable for Santorini plexus or vascular pedicles in laparoscopic radical prostatectomy or cystectomy.

Use of laser in advanced laparoscopic procedures, such as partial nephrectomy, has been reported in animals as well as a small number of humans [14–16]. The advantage of laser is its ability to provide bloodless dissection by coagulating tissue while incising simultaneously. It is also thought to result in less tissue damage than the standard electrothermal technology. However, the use of lasers for hemostasis in laparoscopy remains experimental for the time being.

Overall, these tools can provide effective method for fast and efficient hemostasis. However, the surgeon should be aware of their limitations and disadvantages in order to tailor their appropriate use to each situation.

10.5.1.3 Tissue Sealants

A host of hemostatic adjuncts in the form of tissue sealants are available for the laparoscopic surgeon. Most of the available products are derived from human or animal blood or tissue components, such as fibrin glues, oxidized regenerated methylcellulose, hemostatic gelatin matrix, etc.

As a general principle, all these products do not replace meticulous surgical technique or use of more conventional means of hemostasis.

Fibrin glues contain elements derived from the final steps of the clotting cascade, namely, fibrinogen and thrombin, which are extracted from human blood products and are virally inactivated. The application of these products to bleeding surfaces in laparoscopy is done through a double-cylinder syringe system connected to a long applicator. The two components of the glue (fibrinogen and thrombin) are thus combined in situ to produce the desired hemostatic effect.

Oxidized regenerated cellulose is available in the form of a fleece material that may be applied on surfaces with minimal bleeding to achieve a hemostatic effect. This product is often used in procedures such as partial nephrectomies, where it is used as a sutured bolster to tamponade the defect created in parenchymal tissue following tumor resection.

Gelatin matrix is a two-component product consisting of thrombin and gelatin matrix granula both derived from bovine sources [17]. The gelatin base consists of collagen cross-linked with glutaraldehyde. The two separate components are mixed in a syringe shortly before application, and the solution can be used up to 2 h after mixing. Gelatin matrix can be used in multiple situations during laparoscopic surgery including, for instance, the control of the tumor bed in partial nephrectomy, or to stop bleeding from the neurovascular bundles in laparoscopic prostatectomy.

10.5.1.4 Conclusive Remarks

Several efficient tools are available today for hemostatic control during laparoscopic surgery. Surgeons should be aware of their characteristics and limitations and therefore select them appropriately with regard to their specificity.

For larger vessels of up to 7 mm, LigaSure™ should be preferred, but below 4 mm, all vessel sealing systems seem to be equivalent. Finally, when nerve-sparing surgery is attempted, any device able to provoke thermal diffusion should be completely avoided.

10.5.2 Emergency Management of Hemorrhage

As with open surgery, compression is the first step. Defects caused by laparoscopic instruments are generally small enough to be controlled by the tip of the suction device (Fig. 10.10).

Alternatively, the bleeding vessel may be grasped with a nontraumatic forceps (Fig. 10.11) or compressed using a laparoscopic sponge stick.

In the presence of venous bleeding, some authors recommend to increase peritoneal insufflation pressure. This maneuver has to be weighed against the theoretical risk of a pulmonary gas embolism if the venous defect is significant.

The aforementioned steps will give the surgeon time to analyze the situation and proceed with the best logical approach. In certain cases, compression may be all that is needed to stop the bleeding. Usually, however, more advanced maneuvers may be required.

Finally, conversion to an open approach ought to be strongly considered, especially when the amount of bleeding is unlikely to be controlled by laparoscopic means.

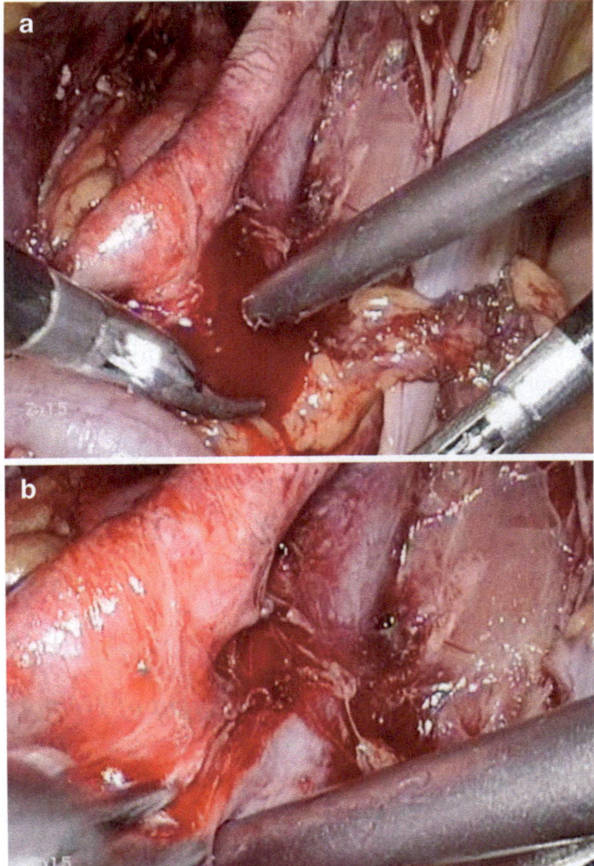

Fig. 10.10 (**a**) Uncontrolled bleeding due to trauma of the right lateral iliac vein. The defect in the vein cannot be visualized due to profuse hemorrhage; (**b**) bleeding is controlled by the tip of the suction device

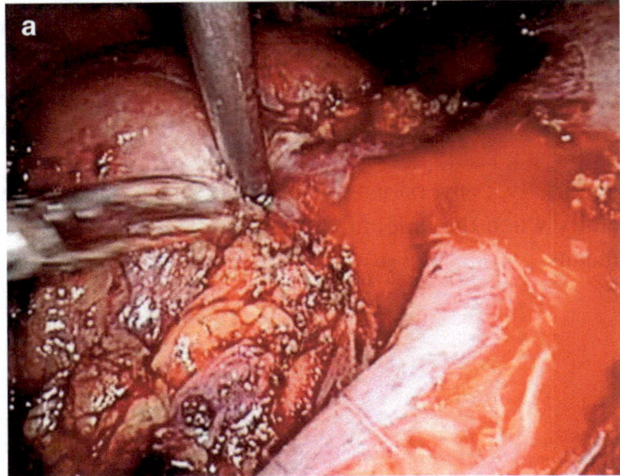

Fig. 10.11 (**a**) Uncontrolled bleeding due to trauma of the right renal vein during a large adrenal tumor resection. The defect in the vein cannot be visualized due to profuse hemorrhage; (**b**) the defect of the vein is clamped with forceps and (**c**) sutured

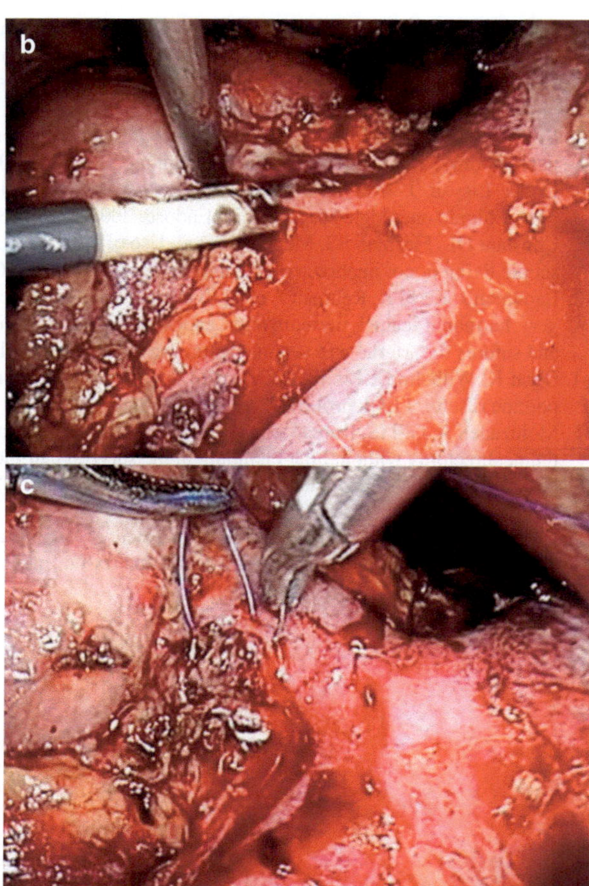

Fig. 10.11 (continued)

References

1. Bazin JE, Gillar T, Rasson P, et al. Heamodynamic conditions enhancing gas embolism after venous injury during laparoscopy: a study in pigs. Br J Anaesth. 1997;78:570–5.
2. Harold KL, Pollinger H, Matthews BD, et al. Comparison of ultrasonic energy, bipolar thermal energy and vascular clips for the haemostasis of small- medium- and large-sized arteries. Surg Endosc. 2003;17:1228–30.
3. Rosenblatt GS, Conlin MJ. Clipless management of the renal vein during hand-assist laparoscopic donor nephrectomy. BMC Urol. 2006;6:23.
4. Friedman AL, Peters TG, Jones KW, et al. Fatal and nonfatal hemorrhagic complications of living kidney donation. Ann Surg. 2006;243:126–30.
5. Hanash KA, Peracha AM, Al-Zahrani HM, et al. Radical cystectomy: minimizing operative blood loss with a "stapling technique". Urology. 2000;56:488–91.
6. Patsner B. Radical abdominal hysterectomy using the ENDO-GIA stapler: report of 150 cases and literature review. Eur J Gynaecol Oncol. 1998;19:215–9.
7. Ramani AP, Desai MM, Steinberg AP, et al. Complications of laparoscopic partial nephrectomy in 200 cases. J Urol. 2005;173:42–7.

8. Chan D, Bishoff JT, Ratner L. Endovascular gastrointestinal stapler device malfunction during laparoscopic nephrectomy: early recognition and management. J Urol. 2000;164:319–21.
9. El-Hakim A, Cai Y, Marcovich R, et al. Effect of endo-GIA vascular staple size on laparoscopic vessel sealing in porcine model. Surg Endosc. 2004;18:961–3.
10. Rosales A, Salvador J, De Graeve M, et al. Clamping of the renal artery in laparoscopic partial nephrectomy: an old device for a new technique. Eur Urol. 2005;47:98–101.
11. Dubuc-Lissoir J. Use of a new energy-based vessel ligation device during laparoscopic gynaecologic oncologic surgery. Surg Endosc. 2003;17:466–8.
12. Constant DL, Florman SS, Mendez F, et al. Use of the ligasure vessel sealing device in laparoscopic living donor nephrectomy. Transplantation. 2004;78:1661–4.
13. Landman J, Kerbl K, Rehman J, et al. Evaluation of a vessel sealing system, bipolar electrosurgery, harmonic scalpel, titanium clips, endoscopic gastrointestinal anastomosis vascular staples and sutures for arterial and venous ligation in a porcine model. J Urol. 2003;169:697–700.
14. Ogan K, Wilhelm D, Lindberg G, et al. Laparoscopic partial nephrectomy with a diode laser: porcine results. J Endourol. 2002;16:749–53.
15. Moinzadeh A, Gill IS, Rubenstein M, et al. Potassium-titanyl-phosphate laser laparoscopic partial nephrectomy without hilar clamping in the survival calf model. J Urol. 2005;174:1110–4.
16. Lotan Y, Gettman MT, Ogan K, et al. Clinical use of holmium:YAG laser in laparoscopic partial nephrectomy. J Endourol. 2002;16:289–92.
17. Richter F, Schnorr D, Deger S, et al. Improvement of haemostasis in open and laparoscopically performed partial nephrectomy using a gelatin matrix-thrombin tissue sealant (FloSeal). Urology. 2003;61:73–7.

Chapter 11
Anatomic Planes and Landmarks in Urologic Laparoscopy

Gyung Tak Sung and Tae Hyo Kim

Abstract The bladder, urachus and medial umbilical ligaments, vas deferens, iliac vessels, and rectum serve as visible landmarks in the transperitoneal LRP. The exposure of prerectal fat shows the proper anatomical plane of dissection between Denonvilliers' fascia and the rectum. An avascular plane underneath the DVC separating the urethra from the DVC must be dissected, which allows the complete identification of the prostate limits and urethra. The following landmarks should be identified in LRC: the medial umbilical ligaments, the peritoneal folds overlying the ureters close to the bladder, the vas deferens on each side (for male), the posterior cul-de-sac of the rectovesical pouch, and the iliac vessels upon initial inspection of the pelvis. The Toldt line, duodenum, and vena cava are important landmarks to expose renal hilum in right radical nephrectomy. The attachments around spleen, descending colon, and splenic flexure are important landmarks to expose the renal hilum in left radical nephrectomy. The psoas muscle is always an initial landmark and serves as a guide for subsequent longitudinal orientation in the retroperitoneal laparoscopic approach.

Key words Urology • Laparoscopy • Surgery • Anatomy • Landmark

11.1 Introduction

Proper understanding of the surgical anatomy is critical in acquiring surgical skills and shortening learning curve needed to perform various advanced laparoscopic procedures.

G.T. Sung, M.D. (✉) • T.H. Kim, M.D.
Department of Urology, Dong-A University Hospital,
3Ga-1, Dongdaesim-Dong, Seo-Gu, Busan 602-715, Korea
e-mail: sunggt@dau.ac.kr

Y.H. Sun et al. (eds.), *The Training Courses of Urological Laparoscopy*,
DOI 10.1007/978-1-4471-2723-9_11,

Herein, the authors will describe key laparoscopic procedures in urology including radical prostatectomy, radical cystectomy, radical nephrectomy, and adrenalectomy.

11.2 Laparoscopic Pelvic Surgery

11.2.1 Laparoscopic Radical Prostatectomy

In the transperitoneal technique, relevant visible landmarks in the peritoneal cavity include: bladder, median (urachus) and medial umbilical ligaments, vas deferens, iliac vessels, and rectum [1] (Fig. 11.1).

11.2.1.1 Posterior Approach

The initial step is a retrovesical dissection of the vas deferens and seminal vesicles. Sharply incise the peritoneum overlying the vas deferens. Divide the vas deferens and trace it distally toward the ipsilateral seminal vesicle, which would be subsequently dissected.

After the assistant lifts the seminal vesicles and vas deferens toward the anterior, make an incision through Denonvilliers' fascia, approximately 0.5 cm below the base of seminal vesicles [2]. Carry the dissection between Denonvilliers' fascia and rectum, preserving the posterior aspect of the prostate and dividing the attachments of the rectum using the blunt dissection tool with suction tip. The exposure of prerectal fat shows the proper anatomical plans of dissection (Fig. 11.2).The lateral extent of this step also serves as an important landmark for antegrade nerve dissection.

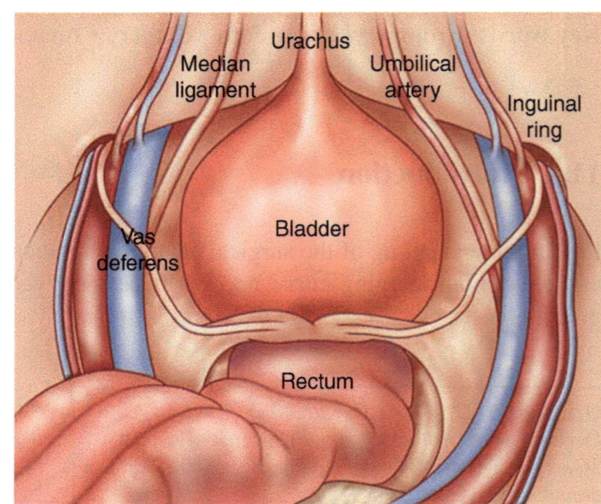

Fig. 11.1 Relevant visible landmarks in the transperitoneal approach include: bladder, median (urachus) and medial umbilical ligaments, vas deferens, iliac vessels, and rectum

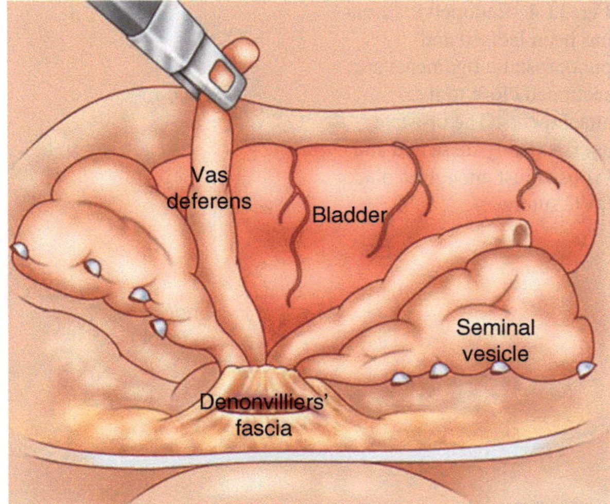

Fig. 11.2 The proper anatomical plane of dissection is shown between the prerectal fat and the Denonvilliers' fascia. The lateral extent of this step also serves as an important landmark for antegrade nerve dissection

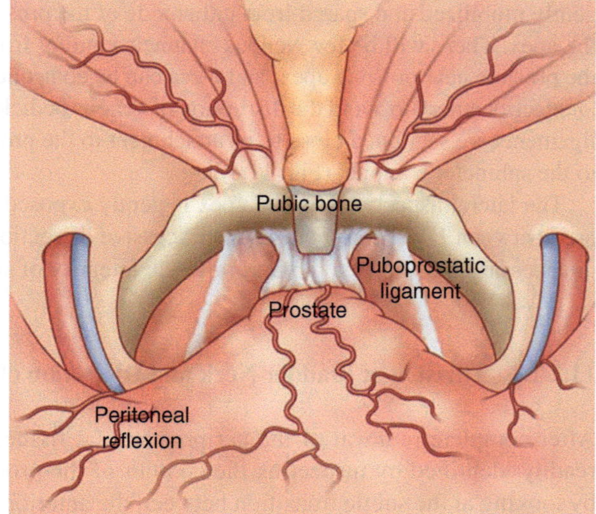

Fig. 11.3 After removing the fat tissues overlying the anterior prostate, visible landmarks are seen and these include: anterior surface of bladder and prostate, puboprostatic ligaments, endopelvic fascia, and pubic symphysis

11.2.1.2 Anterior Approach

The initial step is the incision of median and medial umbilical ligaments above the bladder using a hook electrode device. Applying cephalad and posterior traction on the urachus, prevesical fat is identified, exposing the Retzius space [2, 3]. After removal of the fat tissues overlying the anterior prostate, visible landmarks will show, and these include the anterior surface of bladder and prostate, puboprostatic ligaments, endopelvic fascia, and pubic symphysis (Fig. 11.3).

After exposure of the space of Retzius, the pubic arch is the distal limit for dissection. In a step for incision of the endopelvic fascia, bilateral incisions are performed from the prostate base to the puboprostatic ligaments [2, 3]. Levator ani fibers are

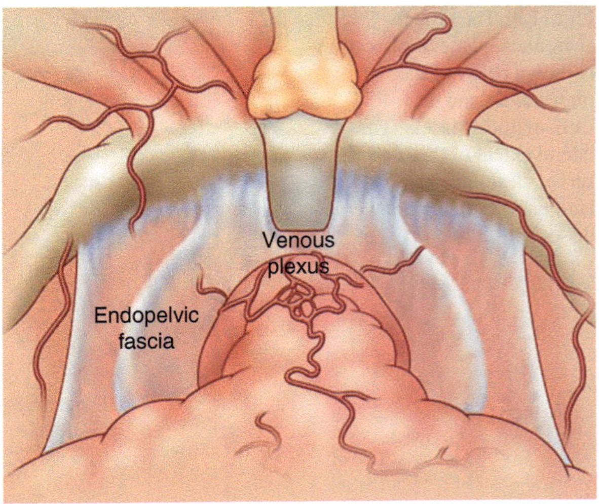

Fig. 11.4 Endopelvic fascia has been incised and puboprostatic ligaments are sectioned close to its attachments. The prostate apex is gently dissected and exposed just enough to place DVC suture

gently mobilized and spared from either side of the prostate, as one marches toward the apex. There will be few venous channels coming from levator ani to the side of the prostate near prostate apex, and these can be controlled meticulously using bipolar electrocautery to avoid the disruption of venous pedicles in the area. Puboprostatic ligaments are sectioned close to its attachment to the prostate sparing its attachment to the sphincter complex (Fig. 11.4).

The lateral aspect of prostate apex is gently exposed just enough to identify the area between DVC and the urethra. Excessive dissection at this area will result in unnecessary bleeding and compromise the integrity of sphincteric complex [4].

11.2.1.3 Division of Bladder Neck and Dissection of the Seminal Vesicles

After complete removal of the periprostatic fat tissues, the proper plane can be readily identified by inspecting the contour of the prostate and bladder neck and by looking at the subtle transition between the anterior bladder neck and the prostate [2, 3].

After judiciously scoring the demarcation line between the anterior bladder neck and the prostate from the midline with monopolar and bipolar electrocautery, the dissection is carried out laterally, freeing the vesical fiber attachments from the prostate. The lateral dissection should not go beyond where venous channels are present at the posterolateral aspect of the prostate (the fat pad of "Whitmore" is the lateral limit of dissection), as it will cause excessive bleeding [5]. The space between the base of the prostate and the neck of the bladder becomes progressively more evident. The anterior bladder neck is incised, and the dissection is continued to find the plane between the posterior wall of the bladder neck and the prostate, while keeping the subcervical urethra – which is completely freed to the level of its posterior wall [5]. The transection of the urethra and posterior dissection into the extending retrotrigonal muscle fibers of the bladder give access to the anterior leaflet of the Denonvilliers' fascia, as the posterior wall of the bladder neck has been completely dissected [6].

11.2.1.4 Dissection of Rectoprostatic Fascia

After the incision of anterior layers of Denonvilliers' fascia, the vas deferens and seminal vesicles are identified. These should be dissected and clip-ligated using minimal cautery. Gentle traction should be applied to expose seminal vesicles. Reliable hemostasis should be applied using clips and bipolar electrocautery as the dissection is carried out closely to the seminal vesicles. One must be careful as not to dissect too widely or excessively use cautery in this area as the neurovascular bundle lies in close proximity to the tip of seminal vesicles [6].

11.2.1.5 Nerve Sparing

The posterior surface of the prostate should be carefully dissected to create a space between the gland and the rectum. This maneuver will create a "trough" under the prostate, which marks the neurovascular bundles at each side (Fig. 11.5). Often, small feeds would be seen from NVB to the prostate on the lateral aspect of the posterior surface of the prostate. These feeds should be meticulously controlled with bipolar electrocautery while staying away from the rectum to prevent catastrophic rectal injury.

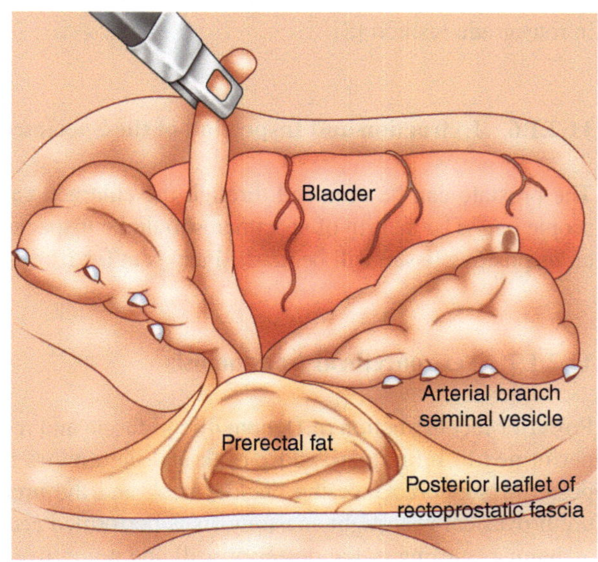

Fig. 11.5 Posterior surface of the prostate should be carefully dissected to create a space between the gland and the rectum. The dissection is carried between Denonvilliers' fascia and rectum, preserving the posterior aspect of the prostate and dividing the attachments of the rectum. This maneuver will create a "trough" under the prostate, which marks the neurovascular bundles at each side

Antegrade Preservation

After exposure of the posterior surface of the prostate from the rectum, the medial border of the NVB is visibly defined. Both the medial border of the NVB and lateral NVB groove serve as critical landmarks to help guide the proper angle and direction of dissection to optimize antegrade NVB preservation. Antegrade dissection starts at the posterior surface of the prostate and proceeds along the posterolateral contour of the gland [6, 7]. Traction for exposure should be carefully applied as to minimize any traction injuries to the NVBs.

There are two key points in nerve-sparing dissection: posterolateral incision of Denonvilliers' fascia and lateral incision of the levator ani fascia [7, 8]. Initial dissection at the prostate should be carried out more toward the anterior at 2–3 o'clock for the right and 9–10 o'clock for the left side of the prostate.

Retrograde Preservation

After ligation and division of the DVC, the urethra is divided at the prostatourethral junction. When incising DVC complex, cold scissors should be used with minimal electrocautery. Excessive use of electrocautery will compromise the sphincter complex. Any bleeding from the DVC can be controlled with superficial stitches under direct vision. Raising pneumoperitoneum temporarily will also reduce DVC bleedings. The prostate apex and the urethra's surrounding sphincter should be meticulously exposed. The urethra is divided step by step using cold scissors, while the muscle fibers of the sphincter and its relations with the apex are visualized. After the urethra is completely transected, the apical dissection is carefully accomplished while avoiding excessive traction. Develop the plane between the levator and prostatic fascia and release the NVBs from the apex toward the base in retrograde fashion [8].

11.2.1.6 Extraction and Inspection of the Specimen

The prostate can be removed through the enlarged camera port site by the endoscopic bag. The margin of specimen should be inspected thoroughly, and the suspicious positive tissue will be marked and sent for frozen section.

11.2.1.7 Vesicourethral Anastomosis

Posterior reconstruction of Denonvilliers' fascia and rectourethral muscle fibers are performed to bring the bladder neck and the urethra more closely and to provide posterior support. Once the bladder neck and the urethra are brought together, a urethrovesical watertight anastomosis is performed according to the van Velthoven technique, starting in the posterior wall and going from side to side until complete anastomosis is achieved [4]. During the anastomosis, Trendelenburg position is lessened, and the pneumoperitoneum is decreased to facilitate subsequent suturing.

11.2.2 Laparoscopic Radical Cystectomy (LRC) in Male

Upon initial inspection of the pelvis, the surgeon must identify the following landmarks: the medial umbilical ligaments, the peritoneal folds overlying the ureters close to the bladder, the vasa on each side, the posterior cul-de-sac of the rectovesical pouch, and the iliac vessels.

11.2.2.1 Mobilization and Division of the Ureters (Fig. 11.6)

The peristaltic ureter is usually visible as they cross over the iliac arteries and dive inferiorly into the pelvis. The peritoneum is incised along the anterior aspect of the ureter and dissected linearly and distally toward the bladder. Adequate periureteric fatty tissue is kept as the distal part of the ureter is circumferentially mobilized. As the dissection approaches near the UVJ, the superior vesical artery and the vas deferens are visualized crossing the ureter [9]. These structures can be either transected or mobilized away from the ureteric surface to obtain maximum ureteric length. The right ureter is then clipped with clips at the UVJ and divided. The distal segment of the ureter is sent for frozen analysis. The distal clip on the transected ureter on the bladder side serves as critical landmarks during the subsequent dissection. The single clip on

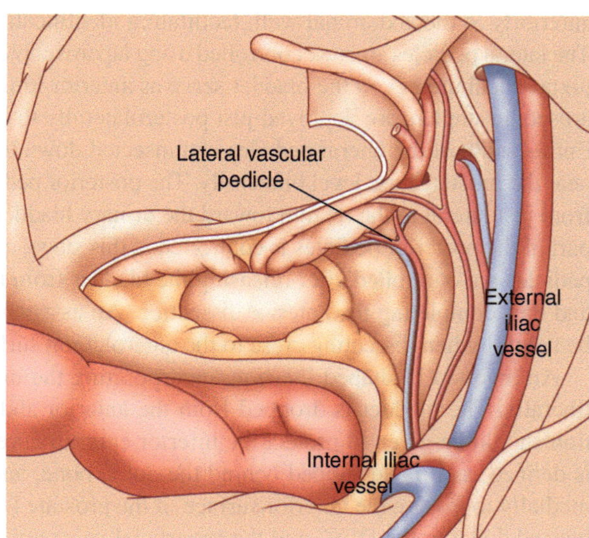

Fig. 11.6 Relevant anatomy in pelvic cavity is shown after right distal ureter has been exposed

the proximal ureter serves to create hydrodistention of the ureter, which will be helpful in subsequent suturing. The left ureter is mobilized in similar fashion. In patients with sigmoid adhesions, adequate lyses might be needed to identify the left ureter.

11.2.2.2 Retrovesical Dissection

As in the posterior approach for LRP, a plane is identified between the rectum and posterior prostate and bluntly developed. It is essential to retract the sigmoid colon proximally to visualize the cul-de-sac. As the ureters have already been mobilized and transected and the lateral peritoneum of the rectovesical pouch is divided, the two lateral peritoneotomies are now joined across the midline [9]. It is important that the peritoneotomy across the cul-de-sac is created distally just 1–2 cm anterior to the surface of the rectum. The plane between the vasa and seminal vesicles and the anterior surface of the rectum is developed. Bilateral vasa and the seminal vesicles are maintained *en bloc* with the bladder while controlling the vessels to these structures [10]. Dissection is continued to expose the posterior layer of the Denonvilliers' fascia, and then, it is incised with cold endoshears to expose the yellow prerectal fat posterior to the prostate. This plane is an important landmark to avoid rectal injury [9, 10].

11.2.2.3 Lateral Dissection and Control of Vascular Pedicles

The parietal peritoneum is incised lateral to the medial umbilical ligaments from the vas deferens at the pelvic brim toward the peritoneotomy across the rectovesical cul-de-sac. The space between the lateral pelvic wall and the bladder is developed by bluntly using suction tip and endoshears, while retracting the bladder medially away from the iliac vessels and the obturator nerve. At this stage, the bladder is still attached anteriorly to the abdominal wall, facilitating identification of bilateral pedicles [10]. The lateral pedicles are now controlled using laparoscopic staplers or clips. Transected juxtavesical ureters on the bladder serve as anterior limit of the resection as the laparoscopic staplers are deployed just posterolaterally to juxtavesical ureters [10, 11]. Entire width of the lateral pedicles is transected down toward the endopelvic fascia, near the prostate base level bilaterally. The posterior pedicles are often seen coursing from just lateral to the rectum toward the urinary bladder. Usually only the cephalad part of the posterior pedicles is controlled at this stage, as caudal part of the posterior pedicles are controlled after releasing the bladder from the anterior abdominal wall, and thus completing the anterior dissection. An assistant's finger in the rectum may be helpful when dissecting close to the anterolateral surface of the rectum.

An inverted U-shaped incision, incorporating the urachus and bladder, is made liberally. The bladder is dropped from the anterior abdominal wall. Careful attention should be given to protect the inferior epigastric vessels. The space of Retzius is defined, as it is developed behind the pubic bone, and areolar tissue is dissected medially to expose the anterior surface of the prostate [10]. The endopelvic fascia is incised down to the DVC, and the superficial veins are coagulated with bipolar forceps and divided. The puboprostatic ligaments are cut with cold endoshears.

11.2.2.4 Transection of Dorsal Vein Complex and Membranous Urethra

The DVC can be controlled with laparoscopic staplers or suture ligation. Often, additional sutures are needed to secure complete hemostasis. The catheter is removed, and the membranous urethra is transected with cold endoshears, after clipping or suture occlusion to prevent local spillage of urine. The remaining posterior attachments of the prostate apex are divided, and the specimen is entrapped in a 15-mm Endocatch bag. To prevent any spillage, the mouth of the bag is double-ligated.

11.2.3 Laparoscopic Radical Cystectomy (LRC) in Female (Fig. 11.7)

After the ureters are clipped and divided, the sigmoid is retracted and the RUMI manipulator (Cooper Surgical, Trumbull, CT, USA) is used to antevert the uterus. The infundibulopelvic ligaments are controlled with either clips or laparoscopic staplers. While the uterus still in antevert and the adnexa retracted anteriorly, the peritoneum over the apex of the posterior fornix is scored transversely with the laparoscopic J-hook [12]. The remaining posterior dissection and vaginal incision is made after preparing the DVC. The lateral pedicles are controlled in usual fashion, and the bladder is dropped. The DVC is suture-ligated. While the uterus is in antevert state, transverse incision of the posterior vaginal fornix is completed at the

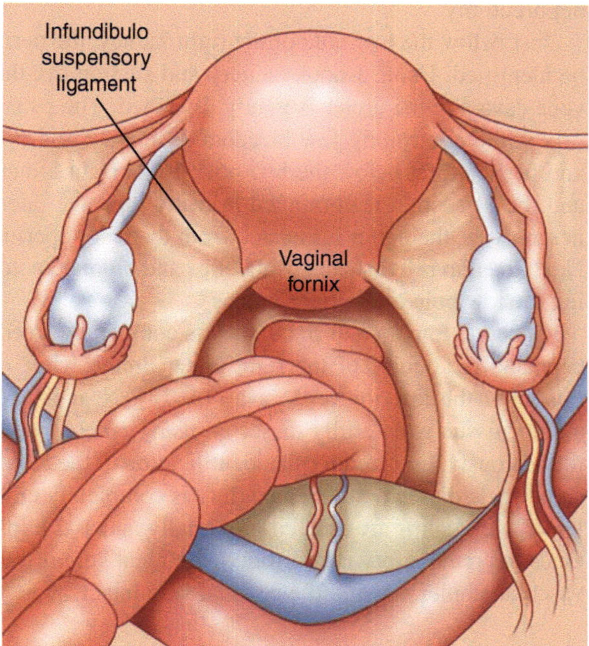

Fig. 11.7 Female pelvic anatomy is shown with the infundibulopelvic ligaments, the uterus, the vaginal fornix, and the sigmoid colon

previously scored site. The vaginal incision is extended distally on either side of the urethra, excising a narrow central strip of vagina en bloc with the bladder specimen. The external meatus and distal urethra are removed using a perineal approach. The specimen is delivered en bloc by the transvaginal route.

11.3 Laparoscopic Abdominal Surgery

11.3.1 Laparoscopic Radical Nephrectomy

11.3.1.1 Right-Sided

The line of Toldt is identified and the colon mobilized. The lateral colonic peritoneal reflection is incised on the right, from the right common iliac artery to the hepatic flexure. During incision of the line of Toldt cephalad, the peritoneum overlying the lateral and upper poles is left in situ, and only the colon is mobilized. The incision is moved medially around the hepatic flexure between the liver and the transverse colon to fully mobilize the ascending colon [13]. In larger renal tumor, the right lobe of the liver may be released from the body wall. The coronary ligament should be incised to expose the upper pole of the kidney, the upper border of the adrenal gland, and the inferior vena cava [13]. The duodenum is identified and then mobilized medially (the Kocher maneuver) until the vena cava and the renal hilum are exposed. In this step, the line of Toldt, duodenum, and vena cava are important landmarks to expose renal hilum in left radical nephrectomy.

Just below the low pole of the right kidney, the peristaltic right upper ureter can be identified. Using J-hook cautery and suction tip, the plane between the inferior vena cava and the ureter is gently dissected. The psoas muscle is identified inferiorly while controlling few bleeders. Using suction tip, the ureter and periureteric and perirenal fat below the low pole of the right kidney are lifted upward en bloc, and the dissection is continued laterally until the lateral attachment of the peritoneum. Now, the ureter is isolated from the rest of periureteric and perirenal fat flap. Next, the flap is transected using clips and bipolar cautery, thus completely mobilizing the low pole of the right kidney.

Once the low pole of the kidney is completely freed, dissection continues along cephalad the course of the right upper ureter, while staying lateral to the medial border of the inferior vena cava [13, 14]. Near the renal hilum, perihilar fibrous areolar tissue is carefully dissected using J-hook cautery. The renal hilum is then meticulously dissected for the identification of the renal artery and renal vein. Using right-angle dissector, the renal artery is completely mobilized to allow clip ligation. Usually 2–3 clips are applied proximally and 1–2 clips distally on the renal artery. Once the renal artery is controlled, the renal vein is transected using the Endo-GIA vascular stapler, leaving the gonadal vein intact.

The remaining attachments of the renal hilar area are freed, using combination of clips and bipolar vessel sealing device. On the medial border of the adrenal gland, the adrenal tributaries are identified on the posterolateral aspect of the inferior vena cava and are judiciously controlled with the Harmonic scalpel. Near the upper medial aspect of the adrenal gland, the inferior phrenic vessels are identified and divided with clips [14]. The remaining attachments of the adrenal gland underneath the liver are controlled with the Harmonic scalpel.

11.3.1.2 Left-Sided

The line of Toldt is incised from the left common iliac artery to the splenic flexure. The incision is moved medially around the splenic flexure, dividing the phrenicocolic and splenorenal ligaments entirely. The colorenal attachments are divided to enable the descending colon and splenic flexure to be rolled medially, as well as dividing the splenophrenic attachments until the anterior aspect of Gerota's fascia and the aorta are exposed [13, 14]. In this step, the attachments around spleen, descending colon, and splenic flexure are important landmarks.

Now, the ureter can be identified along with the gonadal vein just lateral to the aorta. Initial identification and preservation of the ureter facilitates dissection of the lower pole and renal hilum. The landmark for exposure of the ureter is psoas muscle. The ureter lies in the retroperitoneal fat medial to the psoas muscle. Occasionally, exposure of the ureter can be difficult. In this case, the gonadal vessels, ureteral peristalsis, and iliac vessels can be the landmarks to find the ureter [13, 15].

Using endoshears and suction tip, the ureter and gonadal vein are mobilized laterally and superiorly to expose psoas muscle inferiorly. Using suction tip, the ureter and periureteric and perirenal fat below the low pole of the right kidney are lifted superiorly en bloc, creating periureteric and perirenal fat flap. Dissection is then continued laterally until the lateral attachment of the peritoneum. The flap is transected using clips and bipolar electrocautery, thus freely mobilizing the low pole of the right kidney. Once the low pole of the kidney is completely freed, dissection is continued cephalad along the course of the right upper ureter while staying lateral to the medial border of the aorta.

Gonadal vein is mobilized and divided near the renal hilum. It is important not to transect the gonadal vein too closely to the renal vein, as the clips on the distal cut end of the gonadal vein will be in the way of the subsequent firing of the Endo-GIA vascular stapler, for the renal vein transaction. Near the renal hilum, perihilar fibrous areolar tissue is mobilized using J-hook cautery. The attachments cephalad and medial to the adrenal are identified and divided with the Harmonic scalpel. The renal hilum is then adequately dissected for the identification of the adrenal vein, renal artery, and renal vein. Using right-angle dissector, the adrenal vein is mobilized, clipped, and divided. Next, the kidney is retracted in a lateral and posterior direction to expose the renal artery. The renal artery is completely mobilized to allow Hem-o-Lok clip ligation. Usually 2–3 clips are applied proximally and 1–2 clips distally on the renal artery. Once the renal artery is controlled, investing tissues over the renal hilum are lifted and incised to expose the renal vein. The renal vein is then carefully dissected free from surrounding tissue to allow the Endo-GIA vascular stapler. Occasionally, lumbar veins will be seen, but the medial limit of the renal vein transaction usually stays just lateral to the lumbar veins. Remaining attachments of the renal hilum are then controlled while keeping the kidney retracted anteriorly and superiorly. The upper pole of the kidney and the adrenal gland are then controlled with clips and the Harmonic scalpel. The kidney is now completely mobilized in en bloc. The ureter is then identified, clipped, and divided. The specimen is removed intact using Endocatch II bag.

11.3.2 Laparoscopic Adrenalectomy

11.3.2.1 Transperitoneal Approach (Left-Sided) (Fig. 11.8)

The splenophrenic, splenocolic, and splenorenal ligaments are divided using electrocautery. The spleen and pancreatic tail are then rotated medially. The left adrenal gland lies within the perinephric fat at the superior pole of the left kidney. This plane is the landmark to approach to left adrenal gland [16]. The peritoneal dissection is performed until left renal vein is reached. Careful dissection will lead to proper identification of the adrenal gland and vasculature.

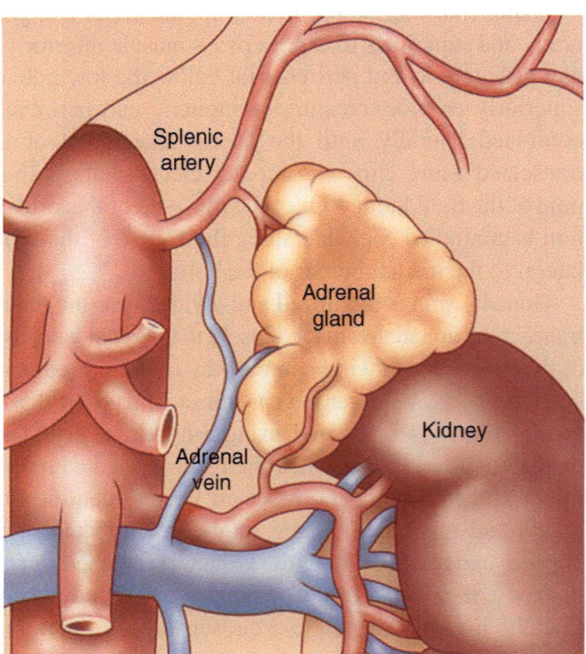

Fig. 11.8 Relevant anatomy of the left adrenal gland and its vasculatures is shown

The left adrenal vein generally descends from the inferomedial aspect of the gland to the left renal vein. It is not necessary to completely expose the renal vessels, for the adrenal vein may be divided near the adrenal gland. The splenic vessels course near the left adrenal gland; the pulsations of splenic artery are an important landmark.

There are generally no specific arteries that need to be identified. The arterial supply for the adrenal consists of an extensive array of small arteries around the medial side of the adrenal that can be easily handled with electrocautery [17].

11.3.2.2 Transperitoneal Approach (Right-Sided) (Fig. 11.9)

For right adrenalectomy, the right lobe of the liver is fully mobilized by division of the triangular ligament. With the liver retracted cephalad and medially rotated, the peritoneum overlying the right adrenal gland is dissected using electrocautery. The right adrenal gland lies closer to the inferior vena cava (IVC) as the left adrenal is to the aorta, which makes this side more difficult. The right adrenal vein usually arises from the posterolateral aspect of the IVC. The exposure of the IVC is a critical step to find adrenal vein from the IVC. The dissection is extended along the medial border of the adrenal up to the superior border of the adrenal gland. After the right adrenal vein is located, it should be doubly clipped and cut. Venous variations may exist, with additional venous tributaries arising from the right renal vein or even the hepatic veins [18]. These veins must not be overlooked during the dissection. As on the left side, simply divide the array of adrenal arteries with electrocautery.

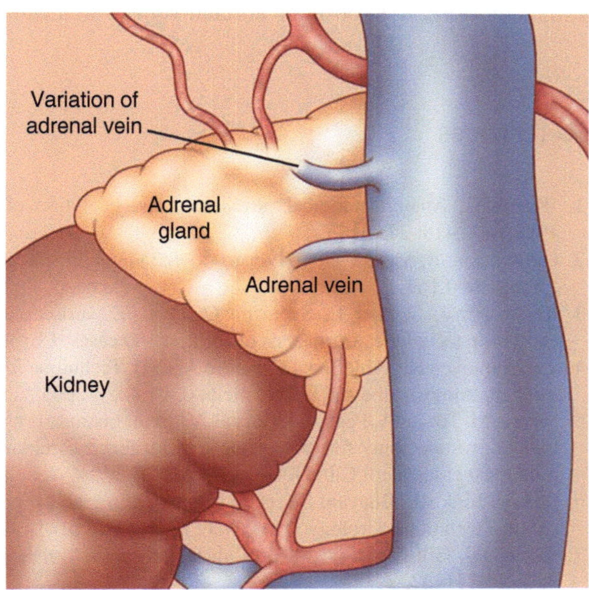

Fig. 11.9 The surgical anatomy of right adrenal gland and its vasculatures is depicted

11.3.2.3 Retroperitoneal Approach (Left-Sided)

The key to the retroperitoneal approach lies in understanding proper anatomical orientation, which is significantly different from the transperitoneal approach. The initial view is always unclear, but key landmarks can be identified. The psoas muscle is always the initial landmark that can be easily seen and serves as a guide for subsequent longitudinal orientation [19].

The dissection is moved cephalad along the psoas to the upper pole of the kidney. The adrenal is approached from a lateral angle, and then, the adrenal vein is exposed along the inferomedial border, where it can be exposed, clipped, and divided. Because the adrenal vein tends to course along the medial aspect of the kidney, the dissection is kept strictly posterior in order to keep the kidney and adrenal gland from falling down into the field of view [19, 20]. After controlling the adrenal vein, remaining attachments of the adrenal gland are detached while lifting and gently retracting the adrenal gland tissue.

11.3.2.4 Retroperitoneal Approach (Right-Sided)

The right adrenal gland is more difficult with a retroperitoneal approach because of the position of the adrenal gland and the length of the adrenal vein in relation to the IVC.

The dissection is moved cephalad along the psoas muscle, taking careful attention to proper orientation. The right adrenal gland rests somewhat more medial to the kidney than the left gland, and the upper pole of the kidney may interfere with the exposure of the gland [20]. Once located, the adrenal gland is mobilized and lifted anteriorly to expose the adrenal vein, which can be controlled with clips.

References

1. Walsh PC. Anatomic radical prosatatectomy: evolution of the surgical technique. J Urol. 1998;160:2418–24.
2. Guillonneau B, Vallancien G. Laparoscopic radical prostatectomy: the Montsouris experience. J Urol. 2000;163:418–22.
3. Rassweiler J, Sentker L, Seemann O, et al. Laparoscopic radical prostatectomy with the Heilbronn technique: an analysis of the first 180 cases. J Urol. 2001;166:2101–8.
4. van Velthoven RF, Ahlering TE, Peltire A, et al. Technique for laparoscopic running urethrovesical anastomosis: the single knot method. Urology. 2003;61:699–702.
5. Menon M, Tewari A, Peabody JO, et al. Vattikuti Institute prosatetectomy, a technique of robotic radical prostatectomy for management of localized carcinoma of the prostate: experience of over 1100 cases. Urol Clin N Am. 2004;31:701–17.
6. Su LM, Link RE, Bhayani SB, et al. Nerve-sparing radical prostatectomy: replicating the open surgical technique. Urology. 2004;64:123–7.
7. Kaouk JH, Gill IS, Desai MM, et al. Laparoscopic orthotopic ileal neobladder. J Endourol. 2001;15:131–42.

8. Simonato A, Gregori A, Lissiani A, et al. Laparoscopic radical cystoprostatecomy: a technique illustrated step by step. Eur Urol. 2003;44:132–8.
9. Basillote JB, Abdelshehid C, Ahlering TE, et al. Laparoscopic assisted cystectomy with ileal neobladder: a comparison with the open approach. J Urol. 2004;172:489–93.
10. Arroyo C, Andrews H, Rozet F, et al. Laparoscopic prostate-sparing radical cystectomy: the Montsouris technique and preliminary results. J Endourol. 2005;19:424–8.
11. Moinzadeh A, Gill IS, Desai M, et al. Laparoscopic radical cystectomy in female. J Urol. 2005;173:1912–7.
12. Clayman RV, Kavoussi LR, Soper NJ, et al. Laparoscopic nephprectomy: initial case report. J Urol. 1991;146:278–82.
13. Caddedu JA, Ono Y, Clayman RV, et al. Laparoscopic nephrecotmy for renal cell carcinoma: evaluation of efficacy and safety: a multi-center experience. Urology. 1998;52:773–7.
14. Gill IS, Meraney AM, Dk S, et al. Laparoscopic radical nephrectomy in 100 petients: a single center experience from the United State. Cancer. 2001;92:1843–55.
15. Winfield HN, Hamilton BD, Bravo EL. Technique of laparoscopic adrenalectomy. Urol Clin North Am. 1997;24:459–65.
16. Terachi T, Matsuda T, Terai A, et al. Transperitoneal laparoscopic adrenalectomy: experience in 100 patients. J Endourol. 1997;11:361–5.
17. Del Pizzo JJ, Schichman SJ, Sosa RE. Laparoscopic adrenalectomy: the New York-Presbyterian Hospital experience. J Endourol. 2002;16:591–7.
18. Chiw AW. Laparoscopic retroperitoneal adrenalectomy: clinical experience with 120 consecutive cases. Asian J Surg. 2003;26:139–44.
19. Micali S, Peluso G, de Stefani S, et al. Laparoscopic adrenal surgery: New frontiers. J Endourol. 2005;19:272–8.
20. Rubinstein M, Gill IS, Aron M, et al. Prospective, randomized comparison of transperitoneal versus retroperitoneal adrenalectomy. J Urol. 2005;174:442–5.

Chapter 12
Urologic Laparoscopic Surgery: Analysis of the Complications

Xin Gao

Abstract Vascular complication during urologic laparoscopic procedures is a rare but most common major complication, which may be due to errors of dissection or access-related trocar injury. A thorough understanding of the anatomy, surgeon's experience, and constant awareness of the potential risks with different kinds of surgical instruments are keys to prevent complications. Prompt recognition and a low threshold for surgical conversion could be lifesaving if a devastating complication occurred.

Keywords Urology • Laparoscopy • Surgery • Complication • Prevention • Treatment

12.1 Introduction

Over the last decade, the popularity of laparoscopic surgery has exploded [1–4]. In China, most of the major medical centers are carrying out laparoscopic operations, and laparoscopy currently represents a primary component of urologic surgery in these centers [2–4].

This has been driven by the potential of laparoscopic surgery to achieve the same goals as a standard open approach while offering the patient distinct advantages in terms of perioperative morbidity, length of hospital stay, and convalescence.

However, there are also disadvantages related to the endoscopic approach. Typically, the learning curve for laparoscopic operations is steep, and there are a number of pitfalls that potentially complicate these procedures. Even for very

X. Gao, M.D., Ph.D.
Department of Urology, The Thirds Affiliated Hospital, Sun Yat-sen University, No. 600, Tianhe Road, GuangZhou, GuangDong 510630, China
e-mail: gaoxin44@vip.163.com

Y.H. Sun et al. (eds.), *The Training Courses of Urological Laparoscopy*,
DOI 10.1007/978-1-4471-2723-9_12, © Springer-Verlag London 2012

experienced open surgeons, it is difficult to translate skills and knowledge directly to the endoscopic technique [5].

Laparoscopy as an alternative to conventional open surgery has been developed rather late in urology. However, it has gained much attention in the last few years due to the patient's demand of minimal access and reduced perioperative trauma while maintaining comparable oncologic and functional outcomes [6].

Although in laparoscopic surgery the approach is minimally invasive, the complexity of the procedure is generally at least equal to its traditional open counterpart. This is also reflected by the range of potential complications, which characteristically encompasses all those already known from open surgery with, in addition, those specific to the endoscopic approach [5].

At present, some laparoscopic/retroperitoneoscopic procedures in urologic surgery, such as radical nephrectomy, adrenalectomy, or pyeloplasty, have almost become the gold standard within a relatively short period of time and with low complication rates.

Others, such as partial nephrectomy, retroperitoneal lymph node dissection, radical cystectomy, and even radical prostatectomy, are highly debated because of the relatively higher complications. Knowledge about these complications is essential for their prevention. Additionally, this understanding helps the laparoscopic surgeon to intraoperatively identify possible complications.

It is the timely recognition which usually allows the surgeon to manage the complication laparoscopically, and thereby preserving the benefits of the minimally invasive approach.

In China, there are many novice surgeons that may lack a specific training in laparoscopy [2, 3]. In this chapter, we aim to focus on the analysis, recognition, management, and prevention of complications that may be encountered in urologic laparoscopic surgery.

12.2 Complications Related to Establishing Pneumoperitoneum

Establishing a pneumoperitoneum and gaining access to the abdomen are the first steps of any laparoscopic procedure. These steps can be challenging and harbor a unique range of complications.

The reported overall incidence of access-related injuries is relatively low. Champault et al. first described the complications related to establishing the pneumoperitoneum in laparoscopic surgery with an incidence below 1% [7, 8].

With increasing experience, over the last decade, complications related to establishing pneumoperitoneum have become less frequent also in urologic surgery [9]. From large series, we can observe incidence rates around 0.2% [10, 11]. However, notably, the mortality rate of these complications has been reported to be as high as 13% [12].

The risk factors associated with establishing pneumoperitoneum are related to the patient's characteristics and the surgical technique. Advanced age, obesity, and wound infection may increase the occurrence of these complications. Of course, the technique used represents the key to prevent these complications.

Advances in trocar design and insertion techniques are ongoing and may further lower the complication rates associated with Veress needle insertion.

Optical-access trocar placement may involve placement of a trocar through a clear blunt-tipped obturator with a recessed knife blade that can be deployed for controlled sharp dissection. Although rare, complications related to trocar insertion with direct vision have been previously reported.

Novel methods at decreasing Veress needle injuries are being investigated. A mesh system placed over the Veress needle to provide facial countertraction during trocar placement has been reported to be associated with no complications [13–15].

12.2.1 The Blood Vessels Injury

As in open surgery, uncontrolled bleeding during laparoscopy represents a major surgical pitfall.

Hemorrhage may occur when gaining laparoscopic access by establishing pneumoperitoneum. In addition, even minor bleeding may jeopardize improved vision during laparoscopy owing to significant light absorption by dark blood staining of the adjacent tissue within the magnified optical field [16]. In these cases, recognition of the complication usually is not a problem. However, in many of the less spectacular complications of trocar placement, the intraoperative recognition of the injury, which is crucial for an optimal management of the situation, represents the main difficulty.

If blood vessel injury from the insertion of the Veress needle is suspected, the needle should be withdrawn and the pneumoperitoneum should either be established by introducing the Veress needle at a different site. Once the camera is introduced, the suspected intra-abdominal needle injury must be verified or ruled out. Injuries caused by the 14-gauge Veress needle can usually be managed laparoscopically even if a major vessel or a parenchymatous organ is involved. If a blood vessel has been punctured by the Veress needle, the bleeding following the withdrawal of the needle is usually not excessive and can be managed by applying pressure for a couple of minutes as well as an oxidized regenerated cellulose and fibrin glue if necessary. Puncture injuries of the near organ can be managed in the same way, or they can be cauterized with the argon beam coagulator. Simple punctures of the bowel or the bladder by the Veress needle do not require any treatment [17].

Successful management of bleeding related to creation of the pneumoperitoneum has opened the field of laparoscopic indications since limitations attributable to insufficient hemostasis or conversion to open surgery related to uncontrollable bleeding has become rare in major laparoscopic centers.

The armamentarium of surgical techniques, instruments, and tissue sealants has significantly expanded. And these advances in hemostasis have been translated into a broader applicability of laparoscopic procedures and a larger diffusion among urologic surgeons.

However, the hemostatic performance and reliability of all tissue sealants used so far are not high enough for surgeons to rely solely on them, and there is no ideal sealant on the horizon. Laparoscopic surgeons must have detailed knowledge of the biophysics of these tools, their spectrum of effectiveness, and their methods of application to perform surgery in a safe manner [16].

Proper knowledge of the vascular anatomy of the abdominal wall as well as understanding of the intra-abdominal anatomy is necessary to minimize the risk of establishing the pneumoperitoneum-related injuries.

Equally important is a thorough preoperative patient evaluation since specific variations of the individual anatomy (e.g., organomegaly, adhesions) can render a patient prone to these complications. Both obese and very slender patients are at higher risk of establishing the pneumoperitoneum-related complications [18]. Previous abdominal surgery significantly increases the risk of intra-abdominal adhesions and bowel injury [19]. In these cases, it is advisable to choose the first entry site as far away from the area of previous surgery as possible. Secondary trocars should always be introduced under direct vision.

12.2.2 Gas Embolism

Gas embolism is a very rare but potentially life-threatening complication. The correct positioning of the needle should be verified prior to carbon dioxide insufflation in establishing the pneumoperitoneum by using a Veress needle. An irregular finding on aspiration, irrigation, reaspiration, or drop test indicates malpositioning of the needle and may lead to the diagnosis of an injury to an intra-abdominal organ. If the intra-abdominal pressure reading at the beginning of the insufflation is not below 8–10 mmHg, incorrect needle position or at least contact of the needle tip with intra-abdominal structures must be suspected and the needle should be repositioned.

It is particularly important to stay in contact with the anesthesiologist during this initial phase. Carbon dioxide may enter the venous vascular system and thereafter be trapped in the right ventricle, causing outflow obstruction from the right ventricle into the pulmonary artery. The initial clinical sign is a drop in end-tidal carbon dioxide concentration and oxygen saturation as well as low-output heart failure, as a result of decreased blood flow in the lungs [20–23].

In case of suspected gas embolism, insufflation should be stopped immediately and cardiopulmonary resuscitation is required. If transesophageal echocardiography is available in the operating room, this may help to visualize the gas embolus in the right heart and make the correct diagnosis. Rolling the patient on to his left side facilitates expulsion of gas from the ventricle. Once the camera is introduced, a cursory inspection of the peritoneal cavity should be performed in every procedure. In case an access injury is suspected, a very meticulous inspection is mandatory to verify or rule out any intra-abdominal lesion. During the past 10 years, we have performed more than 1,000 urologic laparoscopic procedures and have never experienced a fatal gas embolism.

12.2.3 Trocar-Site Hernia

In urologic laparoscopic surgery, trocar-site hernia is a very rare event. However, incisional hernia in 12-mm nonbladed trocar sites have been reported [24, 25]. The most frequent location of trocar-site hernias is the umbilicus, although all trocar sites can be subject to herniation if they are not properly closed.

Trocar-site hernia was first described in 1968 by Fear, who reported this complication after a diagnostic laparoscopy performed to rule out gynecologic diseases [26]. Urologic laparoscopic techniques have contributed to the drastic reduction of incisional hernia, which has traditionally represented a complication associated with open surgery [27].

However, laparoscopic surgery is also associated with a specific type of incisional hernia that occurs at the trocar sites [24, 25, 28, 29]. The incidence of trocar-site hernias is lower than that of incisional hernias after open surgery, ranging from 0.021% to 6%, according to the literature [30]. The incidence of trocar-site hernias also varies according to the type of laparoscopic surgery, with a higher incidence after procedures that require the use of large (diameter more than 10 mm) trocars [24, 25, 27].

Trocar-site hernias can occur 3–5 days postoperatively (early-onset type) and are due to the entrapment of omentum or small bowel in the trocar wound. Therefore, the early-onset hernia is not a true herniation since it lacks a hernial sac and the bowel or the omentum transverse all the abdominal layers, which are open because of an incomplete closure. This can be the case in the so-called Richter's hernia, which presents with exacerbating abdominal pain and small-bowel obstruction due to strangulation of an intestinal loop entrapped in a small trocar wound [31, 32].

When the trocar-site hernia occurs several months after surgery, there is a typical hernial sac, with its content located between the musculofascial layers because of the dehiscence of the fascia. This type of trocar-site hernia is called the late-onset type. The risk factors associated with the occurrence of a trocar-site hernia are related to the patient's characteristics and the surgical technique. Advanced age, sex, nutritional status, presence of anemia, diabetes, obesity, renal insufficiency, steroid therapy, concurrent cancer, and infection of the wound contribute to the occurrence of a trocar-site hernia.

Dealing with a trocar-site hernia is relatively simple in some situations. Factors related to surgical technique include the direction of the skin incision, the lack of closure of some trocar wounds, the technique used for closing the cannula wounds, and the tension exercised on the trocars during surgery. Those related to the surgical material include use of a Hasson cannula, trocars more than 10 mm, trocars with self-retaining collars that need to be screwed into the abdominal wall, blunt radially expanding plastic obturators, and disposable trocars with built-in safety mechanisms and sutures [27, 33].

For those cases of late-onset trocar-site hernias that are not complicated but require surgery, laparoscopic surgery is indicated, especially if the parietal defect is small [34]. In the presence of large trocar-site hernias, open surgery is recommended. A few selected cases of trocar-site hernias can even be treated by placing a polypropylene mesh under local anesthesia. An accurate and complete closure of the abdominal layers as separate layers and an appropriate and correct technique at the time of laparoscopic surgery will undoubtedly contribute to reducing the incidence of trocar-site hernias.

12.2.4 Complications Related to Access in Children

The complications related to access in children are higher because of their special anatomy such as abdominal structures that are more fragile and are closer to the skin [35]. In 1996, Peters reported the first large-scale study of pediatric complications in urological laparoscopic surgery [36]. The study examined reported complications of 153 pediatric urologists during the early years of laparoscopy. Of 5,400 reported cases, there was an overall complication rate of 5.4%, the majority of which were preperitoneal insufflation, subcutaneous emphysema, and herniations.

One of the most common complications related to access is port-site hernia. In the pediatric population, these data are lacking in literature and in Chinese medical literature as well. Waldhausen published a report of an incisional hernia after laparoscopy in a pediatric patient, stating that fascial closure is paramount in all trocar sites 5 mm or greater in infants [37].

As we know, the rates of the complications are most closely associated with the surgeon experience. Additionally, method of port insertion represents also a strong predictive factor, with closed Veress needle insertion being associated with more than twice the rate of major complications when compared to the open Hasson technique (2.55% vs. 1.19%, respectively; $p<0.006$). However, open insertion is associated with a longer insertion time and a higher rate of intraoperative air leaks [38].

Bowel injuries secondary to laparoscopic cannula placement have also been reported [39–41]. Body size affects the rate of injury and complications, as obese children require larger port incisions for proper visualization and insertion. The angle of insertion is also more critical in obese patients, as free mobility around ports is more limited. Conversely, thin children and smaller infants are at higher risk of bowel injury as the abdominal walls are more fragile and abdominal structures are closer to the skin. Other risk factors for injury during port-site insertion include prior abdominal surgeries in the area of trocar insertion, medical comorbidities, anatomical abnormalities, and surgeon experience [35].

Pediatric abdomen is obviously much more fragile than that of an adult. Ports are much more likely to cause inadvertent injury to intra-abdominal structures. The decreased force necessary to penetrate the abdomen is offset by the increased risk of separating the peritoneum from the abdominal wall. This increases the risk for preperitoneal insufflation in children as well as visceral penetration. During procedures involving retroperitoneal approach, the weaker and more posterior reflection of the peritoneum makes it even more prone to inadvertent damage. Additionally, the relative size of the cannulae is much larger in children, increasing the risk of postoperative port-site hernias. Several authors recommend closing all port sites that are 3.5 mm in size or greater [37, 42].

12.3 Vascular Injury

12.3.1 Introduction

Vascular injuries encompass reported complications, such as intraoperative and postoperative bleeding, hematoma, and the need for blood transfusions. These injuries are either access related or occur during dissection [43].

Vascular injuries represent the most frequently encountered complication in urologic laparoscopic surgery. Overall, their incidence rates are low, in the range of 0.7–5.4% [44]. However, transfusion rates (as surrogate marker for vascular complications) have been reported to be as high as 10% [45]. Most commonly, this results from inadequate exposure of the vascular structures, leading to either sharp or thermal injury to the vessel. Additionally, orientation in laparoscopic surgery can be difficult because of a decreased number of reference points as well as a limited field of view, and this may lead to the misidentification of abdominal and retroperitoneal structures.

Both transections of the inferior vena cava [46] and the abdominal aorta [47] have been described as rare complications of urologic laparoscopic surgery. Not surprisingly, the incidence of vascular injuries increases with the complexity of the procedure and decreases with the surgeon's experience. In most cases, these major vascular complications are recognized instantly during the dissection.

In contrast to the former complications, the inadvertent injury to smaller vessels can easily go unnoticed during the course of the procedure. Especially venous lesions can be missed intraoperatively as these smaller vessels do not bleed briskly into the operative field [48]. One important reason for this is the pressure created from the pneumoperitoneum that compresses the injured vein thereby possibly preventing it from oozing blood. These injuries frequently manifest only in the postoperative period when hematomas or hemodynamic instability become evident. Occasionally, blood transfusions or a reintervention is required [49].

Since most vascular lesions occur during dissection, the injured vessel typically is not yet fully exposed at the time of laceration. Locating the source of the bleeding can be a very challenging laparoscopic task. In minor bleeding complications, suction and irrigation may be all that is needed to find the injured vessel, as a trail of blood within the puddle of irrigation fluid will lead directly to the target when the fluid is aspirated. However, if the bleeding is more pronounced, local compression of the respective area is advisable. Through an assistant port, pooled blood in the operating field is constantly aspirated, and as soon as the bleeding discontinues one is sure that the compression is applied to the appropriate site. Under constant aspiration, the tamponade is then gradually removed to reveal the exact location of the bleeding source. If exposure is insufficient, the dissection of the field is carefully continued while pressure remains applied to the lesion. When the lacerated vessel cannot be identified and exposed satisfactorily despite these measures, no further time should be lost and conversion to an open procedure should be performed.

12.3.2 Prevention and Management

One important key to prevent major vascular injuries is a sound understanding of the vascular anatomy in general as well as the vascular anatomy of the specific patient. In this regard, all available radiologic examinations should be carefully studied preoperatively. Especially prior to laparoscopic procedures involving dissection of major vessels, a radiologic examination showing the vascular anatomy in the region of interest should be obtained.

Particularly in laparoscopic surgery with its two-dimensional vision and limited tactile feedback, it is essential to adhere to general surgical principles of a meticulous dissection. Preparation should always lead from the known to the unknown, and no structure should be cut unless it is properly dissected and exposed.

For example, during laparoscopic or retroperitoneoscopic adrenalectomy, the right adrenal vein drains into the inferior vena cava and on the left side the main adrenal vein drains into the left renal vein. However, this pattern shows variations in up to 10%. The most frequent variations are drainage of the right adrenal vein into the right renal vein or into the right hepatic veins. Thus, prior to laparoscopic adrenal procedures involving dissection of major vessels, a radiologic examination, which shows the vascular anatomy in the region of interest, should be obtained and carefully studied.

Some authors suggest access-related vascular injuries should convert to open surgery in order to control the bleeding. According to our experience, some small vascular injuries can be dealt with laparoscopically after all the ports are installed. The range of appropriate measures goes from simple application of pressure to immediate conversion to open surgery. Obviously, the optimal management of an intraoperative vascular complication depends on the severity of the case and the experience of the surgeon. In each individual case, the surgeon must make this decision based upon the respective situation and must choose the solution that least compromises patient safety and the goals of the actual procedure.

The first step in the management of a vascular injury is the application of pressure to the source of bleeding. Effective application of pressure usually requires a small pad or at least sponge gauze to be pressed onto the bleeding site via a laparoscopic instrument (e.g., grasper).

Additionally, the pneumoperitoneum should be increased temporarily up to 25 mmHg to reduce venous bleeding. Pooled blood around the site of the lesion can then be aspirated, and a slow retraction of the pad should reveal the site of the injury.

In minor vascular injuries, application of pressure for a couple of minutes alone may solve the problem. A good option is the additional application of hemostyptic agents like oxidized regenerated cellulose and fibrin glue. Only with adequate exposure of the injured vessel electrocautery or clips can be applied to control the bleeding.

However, in a major vascular lesion, clips, electrocautery, and hemostatic agents usually are inadequate measures. It is important not to lose precious time by attempting to solve the problem with these insufficient measures.

Again, only with adequate exposure of the injured vessel the application of a stapling device might be considered. If the repair of the vessel is vital, laparoscopic suturing of the injured vessel should only be attempted only by the very experienced laparoscopic surgeon.

In our experience, one patient with the injury of an inferior vena cava was sutured by laparoscopic technique during the radical nephrectomy. Usually, additional ports should be placed to optimize distance and angle of the instruments for laparoscopic suturing.

In most cases of major vascular injury, however, it is advisable to quickly convert to an open procedure. The first step should be the compression of the bleeding area with a small laparotomy pad or sponge gauze, as outlined in the preceding section. If a major artery has been transected, however, it may be faster and more efficient to clamp the injured vessel with a suitable laparoscopic instrument. To minimize blood loss and to facilitate locating the injury, it is important to leave the instrument and the tamponade in place until the conversion is finished.

12.4 Injuries to Hollow Organ

Hollow organ injury to the bowel, bladder, ureter, and rectum are frequent complications in urologic laparoscopic surgery. Sometimes, laparoscopic management of these injuries is challenging. Major injury may require conversion to open surgery. In some occasion, an intraoperative or postoperative consult with a general surgeon is recommended, especially for bowel or rectal injuries.

12.4.1 Bowel Injury

The bowel injury incidence in laparoscopic surgery for urologic procedures ranges from 0.4% to 2.5% [50, 51]. Nearly 70% of bowel injuries are not detected intraoperatively and are caused by monopolar electrocautery, Veress needle, or trocar placement.

Pain at a trocar site is a suggestive symptom, especially if associated with diarrhea and flatulence. However, the symptoms may be unusual. Delayed recognition of a bowel injury is a potentially life-threatening complication.

Therefore, it is essential to recognize intraoperatively bowel injuries. However, only one out of three intestinal lesions occurring during a laparoscopic procedure is diagnosed intraoperatively. Patients with delayed recognition of a bowel injury will die as a result of the fatal complication.

The small bowel is the most commonly injured part of the intestine, and therein an injury to the duodenum is associated with the most serious sequelae. Injuries to the colon and the stomach occur less frequently.

Prevention of bowel injuries during urologic laparoscopic surgery seems to be difficult. Experienced laparoscopic surgeons are reported to cause an equal rate of intraoperative bowel lesions as inexperienced surgeons.

Nevertheless, there are recommendations that may help to avoid these rare but dangerous complications. Routine use of a nasogastric tube to empty the stomach reduces the risk of injury to the stomach. Also, preoperative bowel preparation may reduce inadvertent intestinal trauma by increasing intraperitoneal free space and by facilitating operative maneuvers. Manipulation with instruments outside the field of view (e.g., during change of instruments) is prone to inadvertent violation of bowel and other intra-abdominal structures. Likewise, laparoscopic instruments not in use should always be removed from the patient. For the inexperienced laparoscopic surgeon, it is advisable to introduce any new instrument under direct visual control in order to prevent inadvertent bowel injury outside the field of view.

To avoid electrothermal trauma, all laparoscopic instruments must be checked for insulation damage prior to their use. Bipolar electrocautery should be used whenever possible and all diathermy must be avoided close to the bowel. Monopolar electrocautery should not be used to take down bowel adhesions. The lowest possible power setting should be used at all times [52]. The electric energy should only be activated when the entire active part of the instrument is visualized and the tip of the instrument is in contact with the target. To prevent duodenal injury in right-sided renal or adrenal procedures, medial reflection of the duodenum by the Kocher maneuver must be performed using blunt and sharp dissection only. The use of thermal energy must be strictly avoided during this step of the procedure. Innovative instruments such as Ligasure™, which uses a high-current low-voltage output, or the Harmonic Scalpel, which uses ultrasonic energy for both cutting and coagulation, minimize the spread of thermal energy and thereby may reduce the risk of inadvertent bowel injury.

Intraoperatively recognized intestinal lesions can be managed laparoscopically. However, open repair and consultation of a general surgeon should be considered whenever the integrity of the laparoscopically performed repair is questioned.

Another area of uncertainty is the extension of the tissue damage associated with monopolar injuries. Usually, the size of the injury is underestimated. Therefore, whenever an electrothermal lesion caused by monopolar cautery is suspected, resection and end-to-end anastomosis of the involved bowel segment with a safety margin is warranted.

The incarcerated bowel can be managed laparoscopically, if diagnosed early. To prevent this risk, the fascia at all trocar sites larger than 5 mm must be closed under direct vision, ensuring that no bowel could be trapped [53, 54]. High morbidity associated with intestinal complications and the urologic laparoscopic surgeon who is not familiar with advanced laparoscopic bowel surgery should direct the respective surgeon to convert the case to an open procedure or consult a general surgeon [10, 11, 48].

12.4.2 Bladder Injury

Bladder injuries are uncommon in urologic laparoscopic surgery, while they are most commonly reported in association with gynecological laparoscopic procedures [55]. Incidence rates in the literature range from 0.02% to 8.3% [56, 57].

The bladder dome is the most frequent site of bladder injury. In some urologic laparoscopic procedures, such as in laparoscopic simple prostatectomy, opening the bladder dome is needed. Thus, it is easy to deal with the complication. The key step is to determine whether the bladder is injured or not.

If a bladder lesion is not obvious or not immediately recognized, the finding of gas and/or blood in the urethral catheter bag should cause the laparoscopic surgeon to look for any laceration in the bladder. Irrigation of the bladder via the urethral catheter can help to locate the lesion. Once detected, any defect in the bladder wall can be closed with an absorbable single-layer running suture, which most surgeons will be able to complete laparoscopically. Depending on the size of the lesion, the Foley catheter should be left to continuously drain the repaired bladder for up to 10 days postoperatively. An easy and effective measure to prevent intraoperative bladder injuries is the routine preoperative placement of a Foley catheter in all patients undergoing laparoscopic procedures.

12.4.3 Ureteral Injury

Ureteral injuries are common in urologic laparoscopic surgery as well as in gynecological laparoscopic procedures. In a review of laparoscopic pelvic surgery, incidences of ureteral injury between 0.03% and 2% were reported [58].

Clearly, the incidence of iatrogenic urologic injury varies depending on patient selection factors such as history of radiation or the likelihood of retroperitoneal or pelvic fibrosis. The risk of iatrogenic urological injury also depends on the location of the pathology and the extent of dissection required to complete the laparoscopic procedure [59].

The mechanisms of injury include transection, ligation, electrothermal injury, and interruption of the ureteral blood supply. Unfortunately, the majority of these lesions are not recognized intraoperatively, which means that a high level of suspicion needs to be maintained throughout a pelvic or retroperitoneal laparoscopic procedure in order to detect a ureteral injury during the initial surgery.

The most important step toward a successful outcome after ureteral trauma is prompt diagnosis. Therefore, the physician has to have a high index of suspicion based on the injury mechanism and location for this type of trauma to reduce the rate of complications and to perform the appropriate radiographic and intraoperative evaluations in time. If a ureteral injury is suspected, intraoperative diagnosis can be facilitated by the intravenous administration of methylene blue or indigo carmine. Additionally, a retrograde or an antegrade pyelography can help identify the exact location of the lesion. When recognized intraoperatively, laparoscopic repair can be attempted depending on the surgeon's level of expertise.

The key to avoid injury to the ureter is recognition of ureteral anatomy. The ureters course medially in the retroperitoneum posterior to the colon mesentery. Proximal to mid-ureters are immediately lateral to the great vessels and anterior to the psoas muscle. The ureters cross the iliac vessels at their bifurcation and travel posterolaterally along the pelvic sidewall. The ureters then cross under the vas deferens, in men, and the infundibulopelvic ligament, in women, before passing under the obliterated umbilical artery and into the posterolateral aspect of the bladder where they enter via a muscular sheath.

Because of the proximity of the distal ureters to the gynecological organs and rectum, most iatrogenic ureteral injuries occur to the distal one-third of the ureters, particularly in the region of the pelvic brim. When dissecting a ureter, great care must be taken not to interrupt its blood supply.

To avoid electrothermal injury, monopolar current should never be used close to the ureter. Furthermore, routine preoperative ureteral stenting has been advocated in cases where a difficult pelvic dissection is expected [60]. However, some have shown that this measure does not affect the rate of ureteral injuries, even though it might help facilitate intraoperative detection of a respective lesion [61, 62]. This can be regarded as a controversial issue [63, 64]. From our experience, in obviously difficult cases, for example, large malignancies or reoperations, preoperative insertion of ureteral stents might reduce the risk of ureteral injuries.

Dealing with the ureteral injuries is diverse. As in open surgery, the optimal management is related to the location and the extent of the ureteral lesion.

Ureteroureterostomy, ureteroneocystostomy, psoas hitch, or a Boari flap can be performed laparoscopically by the experienced surgeon. It is important to understand that also nonperforating mechanical (e.g., clamping of the ureter) or thermoelectrical ureteral lesions should be addressed immediately. The respective ureteral segment needs to be excised and the appropriate repair done laparoscopically or in an open procedure. In every case of repair, a ureteral stent should be inserted and left in place for 2–6 weeks.

Ureterorenoscopy is a very common technique in China to diagnose ureteral and renal diseases and treat ureteral stones. Since the very beginning, reports of ureteral injury after ureteroscopy have been documented. Nowadays the rate is decreasing because equipment, operative technique, and surgeon's experience have been improved. Ranging from 0% to 28%, the complication rate has averaged at 7% [65].

Depending on the patient's condition, the site, the extent of the injury, and the time of diagnosis, the appropriate management of the ureteral injury must be selected. The type of reconstructive procedure chosen by the surgeon depends on the nature and site of the injury. Ureteroureterostomy, so-called end-to-end anastomosis, can be used for the repair of ureteral injuries to the upper and middle third of the ureter [66]. For extensive injuries to the ureteropelvic junction and the proximal ureter, either pyeloplasty or, if the renal pelvis is severely injured, ureterocalicostomy can be the treatment of choice. For the latter procedure, the lower pole of the kidney must be amputated to expose the infundibulum of the inferior calyx. The ureter is then spatulated and a direct end-to-end ureterocalyceal anastomosis is performed after stent insertion. Ureteral injuries of the distal half of the ureter and an insufficient bladder capacity or other severe pelvic complications can be managed by transureteroureterostomy or transureteropyelostomy. It is a rarely used procedure, which is mainly performed as a secondary or delayed procedure. Injuries involving the lower third of the ureter are best managed by a ureteral reimplantation using a psoas-hitch technique. If the injury encompasses the lower two-thirds of the ureter with a very long defect, not allowing a psoas-hitch technique, ureteral reimplant can be successfully accomplished with the Boari-flap technique.

For complete ureteral destruction, small or large bowel can be used as interposition to bridge the space between the renal pelvis and the bladder. Certainly, this procedure needs standard bowel preparation and therefore cannot be used in the acute trauma setting. It is an operation for secondary repair and should only be chosen if the renal function is relatively normal (creatinine <2.5 mg/dl) [67].

In cases with a solitary kidney and a complete ureteral avulsion, renal autotransplantation can be used to manage the trauma. Nephrectomy is rarely required for the treatment of ureteral injuries. It must mainly be performed when the ureteral trauma is associated with massive renal trauma, for example, in cases of life-threatening bleeding where repair is not possible or severe associated visceral injuries [68].

12.4.4 Rectal Injury

Rectal injuries occur in about 2% of laparoscopic radical prostatectomy, most of them during prostate dissection at the apex. They may result from a direct cut into the rectal wall or from a microperforation secondary to thermal injury due to excessive cauterization on the rectal wall surface [69].

The risk of rectal injury increases when there is a substantial amount of periprostatic inflammatory reaction prior to prostate surgery or radiation, a large volume gland with a narrow pelvis, non-nerve-sparing laparoscopic radical prostatectomy, and surgeon's inexperience.

In the case of surgeon's doubts during dissection, rectal insufflation with air in combination with filling of the operative field with water could prove useful. Formation of air bubbles can be easily detected in the case of rectal injury. Some institutions routinely place an intestinal tube and fill the rectum retrograde with methylene blue or air after prostate removal.

Meticulous dissection is the best way to prevent rectal injury. The principals for treating rectal injury have stemmed from military surgery reports [70]. These principals have traditionally included a diverting colostomy, drainage of the perineal wound, and rectal irrigation. In the case of the untoward event of the rectal laceration, endoscopic correction with two-layer suture must be performed. In a non-nerve-sparing procedure, the perirectal tissue can be sutured and used as an additional layer between rectum and bladder neck.

Parenteral nutrition for 5 days and residual-free enteral feeding for at least 5 days is indicated. Cystography prior to catheter removal should be performed not earlier than 8–10 days after initial surgery. Interposition of an omental flap or pararectal fat flap is not routinely necessary. However, in face of a large, devitalized rectal laceration or of gross soiling, a temporary diverting colostomy is advisable.

Microperforations of the rectal wall often go unrecognized until after the Foley catheter is removed and is manifested by a rectourethral fistula. The first therapeutic option is to reinsert the Foley catheter until the fistula heals spontaneously. If this conservative method fails, elective surgical approach of the rectourethral fistula should be considered.

12.5 Injuries to Intra-abdominal Solid Organ

Solid organ injury to the liver, pancreas, spleen, and kidneys are a known complication in urologic laparoscopic surgery. In a retrospective review of 2,775 laparoscopic urologic operations, the incidences of injury to the spleen, liver, and pancreas were 3.2, 1.1, and 0.36 per 1,000 cases, respectively [44].

Laparoscopic management of these injuries is similar to that described for vascular injury (e.g., increased pneumoperitoneum, direct compression, hemostatic agents, and laparoscopic suturing). Major injury may require splenectomy or conversion to laparotomy.

12.5.1 Injuries of the Liver

Non-access-related injury of the liver during urologic laparoscopic surgery is rare. It may complicate right-sided renal or adrenal procedures and it is usually caused by inappropriate retraction of the liver [71]. Alternatively, a tear in the liver surface can result when adhesions to the liver are strained.

Usually, liver injuries are easily recognized because of the bleeding, although minor parenchymal bleedings may be concealed by the high intra-abdominal pressure due to the pneumoperitoneum. It is therefore advisable to desufflate the abdomen at the end of every laparoscopic procedure and check again for any sources of bleeding.

To prevent liver injuries during laparoscopic procedures, all adhesions to the liver must be taken down carefully at the beginning of the dissection. If the liver has to be retracted during the procedure, the surgeon has to make sure that this is done in a safe and atraumatic way. As long as the respective case and the surgeon's ability allow for it, a retroperitoneal approach can be adopted for another prevention strategy to avoid liver injuries.

12.5.2 Injuries of the Spleen

Injuries of the spleen during urologic laparoscopic surgery are also rare for the experienced surgeon. In the training stage, some tool-related injuries may be observed in the clinical practice. Splenic capsular lesions most commonly occur during the exposure of the retroperitoneum in left-sided renal or adrenal procedures. In recent reviews, iatrogenic lesions of the spleen complicated 0.5–2.5% of laparoscopic and hand-assisted laparoscopic nephrectomies [72, 73].

The majority of splenic injuries during urologic laparoscopic surgery are minor capsular lesions, which usually can be managed laparoscopically. Measures to control these injuries include pressure and the application of oxidized regenerated cellulose, absorbable gelatin sponges, and fibrin glue as well as coagulation with the argon beam coagulator [74]. More extensive splenic lacerations typically result in open conversion and splenectomy.

The key to preventing intraoperative lesions of the spleen is to avoid traction on the splenic capsule. Therefore, any adhesions to the spleen as well as the splenocolic ligaments have to be taken down or incised very carefully during the exposure of the retroperitoneum. Great care must also be taken not to injure the delicate organ with retractors or any pointed laparoscopic instrument, especially when the tip of the respective tool is not in the field of view. If practicable and appropriate, a retroperitoneoscopic approach may reduce the risk of iatrogenic injury to the spleen.

12.5.3 Pancreatic Injury

Pancreatic injuries are uncommon during urologic laparoscopic surgery. However, when occurring, they may represent a devastating complication. Severe pancreatic injury during urologic laparoscopic procedures represents a dangerous event. Large series of urologic laparoscopic procedures have reported general incidences of pancreatic lesions of 0.2–0.4% [5, 75]. Varkarakis et al. [75] found an overall pancreatic injury rate of 0.4% in 890 cases of laparoscopic surgery at their institution. When breaking down the numbers for laparoscopic radical nephrectomies, the percentage of pancreatic injuries increased to 2.1%, with all the injuries occurring during left laparoscopic radical nephrectomies. As described by the authors, surgeries involving the left kidney rather than the right, especially when experiencing a difficult dissection or in the presence of a large tumor, may be complicated by an injury to the tail of the pancreas because of the proximity of this organ to the kidney.

The pancreatic injury may be determined during dissection of massive renal tumor, adrenal tumor, or other urinary tumor. Apart from direct observation, there is no reliable sign that helps to intraoperatively detect a pancreatic lesion.

The prevention of pancreatic injury during urologic laparoscopic surgery again demands solid knowledge of the retroperitoneal anatomy and a high level of suspicion during the procedure. Since pancreatic lesions are commonly unrecognized intraoperatively, the placement of a drain into the surgical bed has been proposed if difficulty with the dissection is experienced in an upper tract procedure. The key to avoiding pancreatic injuries is to completely mobilize the spleen and pancreas en bloc.

Management of the pancreatic injury varies according to the severity of the trauma. When an injury to the tail of the pancreas occurs, management depends on the severity of the damage. If the damage is minimal and the pancreatic duct is intact, a conservative approach can be adopted, with placement of an intraperitoneal drain. However, when the lesion is deep and crosses the midline of the tail of the pancreas, suggesting a lesion of the main pancreatic duct, a distal pancreatectomy must be performed with the use of an endovascular stapler. An intraoperative consult with a general surgeon is recommended.

Unfortunately, the majority of the cases are recognized postoperatively. The patient usually presents with abdominal pain, elevated serum amylase and lipase, and fluid collection on a computed tomography (CT) scan. Management includes complete intravenous nutrition, intravenous infusion of somatostatin (usually 750 mg/day until serum amylase and/or lipase levels normalize), percutaneous drainage of the collection, and placement of a nasogastric tube. Postoperatively, the drain should be left in place until the drainage is less than 50 ml/24 h. Additionally, oral feeding should be withheld until the patient is asymptomatic and has no biochemical evidence of pancreatitis and no evidence of pancreatic fistula.

12.6 Injuries of the Diaphragm and Pleura

12.6.1 Introduction

Diaphragmatic and pleural injuries are rare but are potentially severe complications of urologic laparoscopic surgery. Because of the high intra-abdominal pressure associated with laparoscopy, insufflated gas can enter the thorax through a diaphragmatic lesion and lead to ipsilateral pneumothorax and pneumomediastinum. Injury to the diaphragm during laparoscopic radical nephrectomies has been reported in up to 0.6% of cases [76, 77].

12.6.2 Recognition and Management

Typically a lesion in the diaphragm occurs during the dissection of the renal upper pole. A tear in the diaphragm is not necessarily visible, as electrocautery-induced thermal damage can also injure the pleura. If an injury to the pleura is not directly observed, there are signs of pneumothorax that can be recognized intraoperatively.

In such cases, the use of a J hook should be minimized when dissecting close to the diaphragm because its use has been proven to be associated with higher incidence of injuries to the diaphragm. When the lesion is recognized intraoperatively, direct repair by placement of interrupted sutures should be performed. Care must be taken not to injure the lung during repair. In the event of an unrecognized injury to the diaphragm with development of a clinically significant pneumothorax, a chest tube should be placed and removed after 1 or 2 days.

Although diaphragmatic and pleural injuries rarely occur during urologic laparoscopic surgery, however, they also happen to the highly experienced laparoscopist. There are no specific preventive measures that can be taken to avoid this type of complication. Probably the best prevention is the awareness of the possibility of this injury, especially during the difficult cases of renal upper pole dissection.

12.7 Other Complications in Urologic Laparoscopic Surgery

12.7.1 Lymphocele

Lymphocele is not common in urologic laparoscopic surgery. Lymphoceles occur due to leakage from transected lymphatic vessels. Diagnosis and treatment depend on size, site, and possible infections. Significant lymphoceles may cause pelvic pain as well as voiding problems after catheter removal, leg edema with concomitant pain, deep venous thrombosis, or even hydronephrosis. Infected lymphoceles are often associated with febrile conditions.

Percutaneous drainage, sclerotherapy, or laparoscopic transperitoneal fenestration may be performed [78, 79]. Albqami et al. [80] reported chylous ascites and asymptomatic lymphoceles in 11.9% and 6.8% of patients, respectively. In addition, the Baltimore group reports one case each of transient elevation in serum creatinine and chemical pneumonitis [80]. Stolzenburg et al. [81] performed lymphadenectomy in 389 patients in endoscopic extraperitoneal radical prostatectomy, and occurrence of symptomatic lymphoceles was 3.6%, which is comparable with the existing data on open (extraperitoneal) prostatectomy [82, 83].

The key procedure for prevention of transaction of lymphatic vessels is taking great care to the protection of lymphatic vessels. In our experience, combination of bipolar coagulation, harmonic scalpel dissection, and clipping to deal with the lymphatic vessels can reduce the number of lymphoceles in laparoscopic surgery.

Patients with symptomatic lymphoceles can be managed by percutaneous drainage or laparoscopic fenestration. Access for the fenestration is performed through the periumbilical trocar (mini laparotomy), the site of previous placement of the laparoscope. Generally, lymphocele fenestration requires a transperitoneal approach. In most cases, the lymphocele is clearly visible, and the fenestration is performed starting ventrally and concluding dorsally, taking care not to injure the ureter. If the site of lymphatic collection is not evident, methylene blue can be injected percutaneously into the lymphocele with the aid of ultrasonographic guidance.

12.7.2 Nerve Injury

The obturator nerve is responsible for the innervation of the medial thigh adductor muscles. The obturator nerve injury is rare and can occur during lymphadenectomy by electrofulguration, complete transaction, or entrapment by clips.

When electrofulguration is the cause of injury, the pertaining symptomatology usually recovers after 6 weeks. In the case of iatrogenic nerve transection, some authors advocate a microsurgical epineural end-to-end tension-free anastomosis [84].

Stolzenburg et al. present their data on the obturator nerve injury after their extraperitoneal approach to minimally invasive radical prostatectomy. They encountered a 0.2% temporary obturator nerve apraxia rate, treated successfully with neurotropic drugs and physiotherapy [78]. The same group never experienced complete nerve transaction, which is the same experience as our practice.

Erectile nerve injuries may occur in some patients with localized prostate cancer undergoing laparoscopic radical prostatectomy. The standard technique of nerve-sparing open radical prostatectomy as described by Walsh et al. has produced potency rates of 60–76% [85, 86]. The preservation of erectile nerve following radical prostatectomy for localized prostate cancer is an important and often achievable goal.

Better understanding of the relevant anatomy and improvements in surgical technique has led to much greater preservation of erectile function and no injury of the erectile nerve post-laparoscopic radical prostatectomy.

Other nerve injury due to intraoperative positioning is caused by stretch, ischemia, or compression. Risk factors include thin body habitus, diabetes mellitus, existing neuropathy, peripheral vascular disease, malnutrition, and intraoperative hypothermia or hypotension. Particular care should be taken, especially in high-risk patients, to properly pad and position [87].

References

1. Gao X, Pang J, Li LY, et al. Expression profiling identifies new function of collapsin response mediator protein 4 as a metastasis-suppressor in prostate cancer. Oncogene. 2010;29: 4555–66.
2. Gao X, Wang KB, Pu XY, et al. Modified apical dissection of the prostate improves early continence in laparoscopic radical prostatectomy: technique and initial results. J Cancer Res Clin Oncol. 2009;136:511–6.
3. Gao X, Zhou JH, Li LY, et al. Laparoscopic radical prostatectomy: oncological and functional results of 126 patients with a minimum 3-year follow-up at a single Chinese institute. Asian J Androl. 2009;11(5):548–56.
4. Pu XY, Wang XH, Wu YL, et al. Comparative study of the impact of 3- versus 8-month neoadjuvant hormonal therapy on outcome of laparoscopic radical prostatectomy. J Cancer Res Clin Oncol. 2007;133:555–62.
5. Muntener M, Romero RF, Kavoussi LR. Complications in laparoscopic surgery. In: Hohenfellner M, Santucci R, editors. Emergencies in urology. Berlin, Heidelberg: Springer; 2007.

6. Burchardt M, Stolzenburg JU. Complications in laparoscopic urology. World J Urol. 2008;26:521–2.
7. Champault G, Cazacu F. Laparoscopic surgery: injuries caused by trocars (French Survey 1994) in reference to 103,852 interventions. J Chir. 1995;132:109–13.
8. Champault G, Cazacu F, Taffinder N. Serious trocar accidents in laparoscopic surgery: a French survey of 103,852 operations. Surg Laparosc Endosc. 1996;6:367–70.
9. Gettman MT. Complications of laparoscopic access. In: Ramakumar S, Jarrett T, editors. Complications of urologic laparoscopic surgery. Boca Raton: Taylor& Francis; 2005.
10. Clayman RV. Multi-institutional study of complications in 1085 laparoscopic urologic procedures. J Urol. 2002;168:871–2.
11. Soulie M, Salomon L, Seguin P, et al. Multi-institutional study of complications in 1085 laparoscopic urologic procedures. Urology. 2001;58:899–903.
12. Chandler JG, Corson SL, Way LW. Three spectra of laparoscopic entry access injuries. J Am Coll Surg. 2001;192:478–90; discussion 490–71.
13. Clayman RV. Radially expanding laparoscopic access for renal/adrenal surgery. J Urol. 2002;168:872–3.
14. Lam TY, Lee SW, So HS, et al. Radially expanding trocar: a less painful alternative for laparoscopic surgery. J Laparoendosc Adv Surg Tech. 2000;10:269–73.
15. Shekarriz B, Gholami SS, Rudnick DM, et al. Radially expanding laparoscopic access for renal/adrenal surgery. Urology. 2001;58:683–7.
16. Klingler CH, Remzi M, Marberger M, et al. Haemostasis in laparoscopy. Eur Urol. 2006;50:948–56; discussion 956–47.
17. Gill IS, Meraney AM, Clayman RV. Basic principles techniques, and equipment of laparoscopic surgery. In: Walsh PC, Retik AB, Vaughan Jr ED, et al., editors. Campbell's urology. 8th ed. Philadelphia: Saunders; 2002.
18. Chapron CM, Pierre F, Lacroix S, et al. Major vascular injuries during gynecologic laparoscopy. J Am Coll Surg. 1997;185:461–5.
19. Lecuru F, Leonard F, Philippe Jais J, et al. Laparoscopy in patients with prior surgery: results of the blind approach. JSLS. 2001;5:13–6.
20. Beck DH, McQuillan PJ. Fatal carbon dioxide embolism and severe haemorrhage during laparoscopic salpingectomy. Br J Anaesth. 1994;72:243–5.
21. Blaser A, Rosset P. Fatal carbon dioxide embolism as an unreported complication of retroperitoneoscopy. Surg Endosc. 1999;13:713–4.
22. de Plater RM, Jones IS. Non-fatal carbon dioxide embolism during laparoscopy. Anaesth Intensive Care. 1989;17:359–61.
23. Lantz PE, Smith JD. Fatal carbon dioxide embolism complicating attempted laparoscopic cholecystectomy-case report and literature review. J Forensic Sci. 1994;39:1468–80.
24. Kouba EJ, Hubbard JS, Wallen E, et al. Incisional hernia in a 12-mm nonbladed trocar site following laparoscopic nephrectomy. Scientific World Journal. 2006;6:2399–402.
25. Kouba EJ, Hubbard JS, Wallen E, et al. Incisional hernia in a 12-mm non-bladed trocar site following laparoscopic nephrectomy. Urol Int. 2007;79:276–9.
26. Fear RE. Laparoscopy a valuable aid in gynecologic diagnosis. ISRN Obstet Gynecol. 1968;31:297–309.
27. Chiu CC, Lee WJ, Wang W, et al. Prevention of trocar-wound hernia in laparoscopic bariatric operations. Obes Surg. 2006;16:913–8.
28. Hussain A, Mahmood H, Shuaib S, et al. Prevention of trocar site incisional hernia following laparoscopic ventral hernia repair. JSLS. 2008;12:206–9.
29. Uslu HY, Erkek AB, Cakmak A, et al. Trocar site hernia after laparoscopic cholecystectomy. J Laparoendosc Adv Surg Tech A. 2007;17:600–3.
30. Bartone G, Crovella F. Trocar-site hernia. In: Crovella F, Bartone G, Fei L, editors. Incisional hernia. Milano: Springer Milan; 2008.
31. Bendsen AK, Bauer T, Johansen TP. Richter hernia in trocar site after laparoscopic herniotomy. Ugeskr Laeger. 1995;157:6438–9.

32. Matthews BD, Heniford BT, Sing RF. Preperitoneal Richter hernia after a laparoscopic gastric bypass. Surg Laparosc Endosc Percutan Tech. 2011;11:47–9.
33. Eid GM, Collins J. Application of a trocar wound closure system designed for laparoscopic procedures in morbidly obese patients. Obes Surg. 2005;15:871–3.
34. Susmallian S, Ezri T, Charuzi I. Laparoscopic repair of access port site hernia after Lap-Band system implantation. Obes Surg. 2002;12:682–4.
35. Akhavan A, Stock JA. Complications and management of pediatric robotic-assisted laparoscopic surgery: prevention and management. In: Palmer JS, editor. Current clinical urology: pediatric robotic urology. New York: Humana Press; 2009.
36. Peters CA. Complications in pediatric urological laparoscopy: results of a survey. J Urol. 1996;155:1070–3.
37. Waldhaussen JH. Incisional hernia in a 5-mm trocar site following pediatric laparoscopy. J Laparoendosc Surg. 1996;6 Suppl 1:S89–90.
38. Bemelman WA, Dunker MS, Busch OR, et al. Efficacy of establishment of pneumoperitoneum with the Veress needle, Hasson trocar, and modified blunt trocar (TrocDoc): a randomized study. J Laparoendosc Adv Surg Tech A. 2000;10:325–30.
39. El-Banna M, Abdel-Atty M, El-Meteini M, et al. Management of laparoscopic-related bowel injuries. Surg Endosc. 2000;14:779–82.
40. Schrenk P, Woisetschlager R, Rieger R, et al. Mechanism, management, and prevention of laparoscopic bowel injuries. Gastrointest Endosc. 1996;43:572–4.
41. Vilos GA. Laparoscopic bowel injuries: forty litigated gynaecological cases in Canada. J Obstet Gynaecol Can. 2002;24:224–30.
42. Bloom DA, Ehrlich RM. Omental evisceration through small laparoscopy port sites. J Endourol. 1993;7:31–2; discussion 32–3.
43. Fahlenkamp D, Rassweiler J, Fornara P, et al. Complications of laparoscopic procedures in urology: experience with 2,407 procedures at 4 German centers. J Urol. 1999;162:765–70; discussion 770–61.
44. Permpongkosol S, Link RE, Su LM, et al. Complications of 2,775 urological laparoscopic procedures: 1993 to 2005. J Urol. 2007;177:580–5.
45. Emeriau D, Vallee V, Tauzin-Fin P, et al. Morbidity of unilateral and bilateral laparoscopic adrenalectomy according to the indication. Report of a series of 100 consecutive cases. Prog Urol. 2005;15:626–31.
46. McAllister M, Bhayani SB, Ong A, et al. Vena caval transection during retroperitoneoscopic nephrectomy: report of the complication and review of the literature. J Urol. 2004;172:183–5.
47. Sautter T, Haueisen H, Stierli P, et al. A severe complication of retroperitoneoscopic nephrectomy. J Urol. 2001;165:515–6.
48. Strebel RT, Muntener M, Sulser T. Intraoperative complications of laparoscopic adrenalectomy. World J Urol. 2008;26:555–60.
49. Rosevear HM, Montgomery JS, Roberts WW, et al. Characterization and management of postoperative hemorrhage following upper retroperitoneal laparoscopic surgery. J Urol. 2006;176:1458–62.
50. Gill IS, Clayman RV, Albala DM, et al. Retroperitoneal and pelvic extraperitoneal laparoscopy: an international perspective. Urology. 1998;52:566–71.
51. Bishoff JT, Allaf ME, Kirkels W, et al. Laparoscopic bowel injury: incidence and clinical presentation. J Urol. 1999;161:887–90.
52. Saye WB, Miller W, Hertzmann P. Electrosurgery thermal injury. Myth or misconception? Surg Laparosc Endosc. 1991;1:223–8.
53. Parra RO, Hagood PG, Boullier JA, et al. Complications of laparoscopic urological surgery: experience at St. Louis University. J Urol. 1994;151:681–4.
54. Soulie M, Seguin P, Richeux L, et al. Urological complications of laparoscopic surgery: experience with 350 procedures at a single center. J Urol. 2001;165:1960–3.

55. Hasson HM, Parker WH. Prevention and management of urinary tract injury in laparoscopic surgery. J Am Assoc Gynecol Laparosc. 1998;5:99–114.
56. Jelovsek JE, Chiung C, Chen G, et al. Incidence of lower urinary tract injury at the time of total laparoscopic hysterectomy. JSLS. 2007;11:422–7.
57. Vakili B, Chesson RR, Kyle BL, et al. The incidence of urinary tract injury during hysterectomy: a prospective analysis based on universal cystoscopy. Am J Obstet Gynecol. 2005;192:1599–604.
58. Ostrzenski A, Radolinski B, Ostrzenska KM. A review of laparoscopic ureteral injury in pelvic surgery. Obstet Gynecol Surv. 2003;58:794–9.
59. Chen RN. Avoidance and treatment of urological complications. In: MacFadyen Jr BV, Arregui ME, Eubanks S, et al., editors. Laparoscopic surgery of the abdomen. New York: Springer; 2004.
60. Leff EI, Groff W, Rubin RJ, et al. Use of ureteral catheters in colonic and rectal surgery. Dis Colon Rectum. 1982;25:457–60.
61. Bothwell WN, Bleicher RJ, Dent TL. Prophylactic ureteral catheterization in colon surgery. A five-year review. Dis Colon Rectum. 1994;37:330–4.
62. Kuno K, Menzin A, Kauder HH, et al. Prophylactic ureteral catheterization in gynecologic surgery. Urology. 1998;52:1004–8.
63. Chou MT, Wang CJ, Lien RC. Prophylactic ureteral catheterization in gynecologic surgery: a 12-year randomized trial in a community hospital. Int Urogynecol J Pelvic Floor Dysfunct. 2009;20:689–93.
64. Peters WA. Intraoperative ureteral catheterization through a cystotomy: an adjuvant in gynecologic surgery. South Med J. 1982;75:1400–2.
65. McAninch JW, Santucci RA. Genitourinary trauma. In: Walsh PC, Retik AB, Vaughan Jr ED, et al., editors. Campbell's urology. 8th ed. Philadelphia: Saunders; 2002.
66. Lynch TH, Martinez-Pineiro L, Plas E, et al. EAU guidelines on urological trauma. Eur Urol. 2005;47:1–15.
67. Armenakas NA. Current methods of diagnosis and management of ureteral injuries. World J Urol. 1999;17:78–83.
68. McGinty DM, Mendez R. Traumatic ureteral injuries with delayed recognition. Urology. 1997;10:115–7.
69. Lampert R, Weih EH, Breucking E, et al. Postoperative bilateral compartment syndrome resulting from prolonged urological surgery in lithotomy position. Serum creatine kinase activity (CK) as a warning signal in sedated, artificially respirated patients. Der Anaesthesist. 1995;44:43–7.
70. Ganchrow MI, Lavenson Jr GS, et al. Surgical management of traumatic injuries of the colon and rectum. Arch Surg. 1970;100:515–20.
71. Ogan K, Cadeddu JA. Liver injury during urologic laparoscopy. In: Ramakumar S, Jarrett T, editors. Complications of urologic laparoscopic surgery. Boca Raton: Taylor& Francis; 2005.
72. Hedican SP. Complications of hand-assisted laparoscopic urologic surgery. J Endourol. 2004;18:387–96.
73. Melcher ML, Carter JT, Posselt A, et al. More than 500 consecutive laparoscopic donor nephrectomies without conversion or repeated surgery. Arch Surg. 2005;140:835–9; discussion 839–40.
74. Canby-Hagino ED, Morey AF, Jatoi I, et al. Fibrin sealant treatment of splenic injury during open and laparoscopic left radical nephrectomy. J Urol. 2000;164:2004–5.
75. Varkarakis IM, Allaf ME, Bhayani SB, et al. Pancreatic injuries during laparoscopic urologic surgery. Urology. 2004;64:1089–93.
76. Aron M, Colombo Jr JR, Turna B, et al. Diaphragmatic repair and/or reconstruction during upper abdominal urological laparoscopy. J Urol. 2007;178:2444–50.
77. Del Pizzo JJ, Jacobs SC, Bishoff JT, et al. Pleural injury during laparoscopic renal surgery: early recognition and management. J Urol. 2003;169:41–4.

78. Stolzenburg JU, Rabenalt R, Do M, et al. Complications of endoscopic extraperitoneal radical prostatectomy (EERPE): prevention and management. World J Urol. 2006;24:668–75.
79. Stolzenburg JU, Rabenalt R, Do M, et al. Categorisation of complications of endoscopic extraperitoneal and laparoscopic transperitoneal radical prostatectomy. World J Urol. 2006;24:88–93.
80. Albqami N, Janetschek G. Laparoscopic retroperitoneal lymph-node dissection in the management of clinical stage I and II testicular cancer. J Endourol. 2005;19:683–92; discussion 692.
81. Permpongkosol S, Lima GC, Warlick CA, et al. Postchemotherapy laparoscopic retroperitoneal lymph node dissection: evaluation of complications. Urology. 2007;69:361–5.
82. Van Velthoven RF. Laparoscopic radical prostatectomy: transperitoneal versus retroperitoneal approach: is there an advantage for the patient? Curr Opin Urol. 2005;15:83–8.
83. Martina GR, Giumelli P, Scuzzarella S, et al. Laparoscopic extraperitoneal radical prostatectomy–learning curve of a laparoscopy-naive urologist in a community hospital. Urology. 2005;65:959–63.
84. Spaliviero M, Steinberg AP, Kaouk JH, et al. Laparoscopic injury and repair of obturator nerve during radical prostatectomy. Urology. 2004;64:1030.
85. Quinlan DM, Epstein JI, Carter BS, et al. Sexual function following radical prostatectomy: influence of preservation of neurovascular bundles. J Urol. 1991;145:998–1002.
86. Kundu SD, Roehl KA, Eggener SE, et al. Potency, continence and complications in 3,477 consecutive radical retropubic prostatectomies. J Urol. 2004;172:2227–31.
87. Winfree CJ, Kline DG. Intraoperative positioning nerve injuries. Surg Neurol. 2005;63:5–18; discussion 18.

Index

Y.H. Sun et al. (eds.), *The Training Courses of Urological Laparoscopy*,
DOI 10.1007/978-1-4471-2723-9, © Springer-Verlag London 2012

L

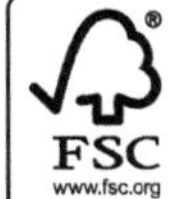

MIX
Papier aus verantwortungsvollen Quellen
Paper from responsible sources
FSC® C105338

If you have any concerns about our products,
you can contact us on
ProductSafety@springernature.com

In case Publisher is established outside the EU,
the EU authorized representative is:
Springer Nature Customer Service Center GmbH
Europaplatz 3, 69115 Heidelberg, Germany

Printed by Libri Plureos GmbH
in Hamburg, Germany